MW01130845

"For way too long the glo
us nowhere because we
magnitude of the problem. Over the p
to the recognition of self-responsibility, to go beyond overwhelm —
possibility step-by-step. Climate change is undoubtedly a global challenge, but in
addressing it we are learning about ourselves as individual members of society. We
are learning about our still only partially unleashed potential for good. In her unique
style, Leslie Davenport takes us through this remarkable journey of self and planet."

*—Christiana Figueres, former Executive Secretary of
the UN Convention on Climate Change*

"Breaking new ground with healing responses to climate chaos, Leslie Davenport
brings not only abundant psychological methodology, but also deep ecological
wisdom. This is a book of rare significance. Extending far beyond a 'clinician's guide,'
it recognizes that climate change and action let us experience our unity with all life,
and serve as catalyst for collective transformation."

—Joanna Macy, author of Coming Back to Life: The
Updated Guide to the Work that Reconnects

"As we enter this revolutionary time on the planet, Leslie Davenport breaks new ground
in synthesizing climate science, conscious self-awareness of our interconnectedness
with all species and the living earth, ecological psychology, and deep resiliency
practices that provide practical guidance for a sustainable future. While it is an
excellent textbook, the accessible tone makes it an essential read for anyone seeking
insight, inspiration, and a path for effective engagement."

*—Brian Thomas Swimme, Professor of Cosmology at the
California Institute of Integral Studies, and author of* The Hidden
Heart of the Cosmos: Humanity and the New Story

"In an era of climate change and climate denial, all of us need ways to connect to the
people and resources that will make us more resilient to challenges. This focused,
deeply passionate book provides us with the tools that we all need to recognize the
impediments to resilient action and create lives where we can connect with each other
and our environment in ways that improve and nurture them. Using a mix of actual
disaster cases, applied exercises, and theory, this book sets the bar for the field."

*—Daniel P. Aldrich, Professor and Director of the Security and Resilience
Studies program at NEU and author of* Building Resilience

"This book is essential reading for anyone motivated by healing and increasing
resiliency among individuals and communities in this time of increasingly turbulent
change. Drawing the essential connections between human trauma and large-scale
events as Earth's ecological systems are in serious and accelerating decline, Leslie
presents, in accessible and compelling ways, the data and experiential practices that
can allow us to approach the emotional and psychological impacts of living during
the Great Turning feeling resourced and with some equilibrium ourselves. Given the
scale and depth of the challenges we face and their enduring impacts on people, this
book is an invaluable resource for all who care about engaging with each other and
the world consciously in this pivotal time."

—Nina Simons, Co-Founder and President, Bioneers

"If you despair for the future of this planet, if you worry about the state of our collective common sense, read this book. MIT's Peter Senge once told me that the success of an intervention is determined by the inner condition of the intervener. Leslie Davenport's work overflows with valuable advice and tools for a healthier inner ecology. This powerful, important book should be on the bedside table of every climate intervener."

—*James Hoggan, Founder of DeSmogBlog and author of* Climate Cover-Up

"Leslie Davenport has created an invaluable resource for anyone wanting to address climate change effectively and wisely. *Emotional Resiliency* shines a light on the psychological underpinnings that thwart climate progress, and provides tools for meaningful conversations and creative solutions. She reconnects us to the essence of our humanity as part of the diverse web of life. There are a wealth of practices that support an ecoharmonious lifestyle and courageous resiliency for promoting change from personal to policy levels. This book is a hopeful light and a practical asset for navigating the challenges of climate work."

—*Lynne Twist, Co-Founder of Pachamama Alliance*

"We know it's no longer enough to simply unleash more startling facts and blast images of our planet being violated. We also need to cultivate a pragmatic form of hope by helping develop empowering actions, a clear direction, ways to connect with collective and systemic support, practices for effective self-care, and the tools and methods necessary for change. By taking a dive into the prospects and practices that this book offers, we will all learn to do just that."

—*Lise Van Susteren, M.D., Climate Energy and Environmental Committee of the Metropolitan Washington Council of Governments in Washington, DC*

"Psychology has given us the tools to help us through the stages of personal grief, but now there is a vital need to help us navigate the collective grief of our present ecocide, the depletion of species, the destruction of our ecosystem. Leslie Davenport gives us a grounded perspective on what climate change means to our body and our psyche, and simple practices to make the inner and outer changes we need to reconnect with the nurturing Earth and its deep life-sustaining energy. She helps us to find true resiliency—a much-needed handbook for these challenging times."

—*Llewellyn Vaughan-Lee, author of* Spiritual Ecology

"Although we are familiar with the physical impacts of climate change, Leslie Davenport argues, with great prescience, that we have too long ignored the deeper psychological impacts. Her book is invaluable: both for the light it throws on why climate change is so hard for us to accept and as a manual for how we can learn to cope and adapt to the growing threats to our sense of place and identity."

—*George Marshall, Founder of Climate Outreach and author of* Don't Even Think About It: Why Our Brains Are Wired to Ignore Climate Change

"The symptoms of the planet are appearing in the consulting room. Grief, anxiety, and depression can no longer be relegated solely to the interior of the patient. And more, these same conditions are befalling therapists as well. *Emotional Resiliency in the Era of Climate Change* offers a therapy which touches the circumstances of our rapidly changing environment. Unflinching in its examination of our current ecological crisis yet suffused with a seasoned wisdom that offers more than hope; it grants a vision of a psyche attuned to the pulse of the living world. And isn't this what we need in this late hour? Davenport's intelligent, compassionate book is both timely and essential. It is filled with the perspectives and practices which enable us to respond to our dire times with a greater capacity for meaningful change. A vital and needed work."

—*Francis Weller, author of* The Wild Edge of Sorrow:
Rituals of Renewal and the Sacred Work of Grief

"Mental health professionals have been slow to move beyond individualistic paradigms of mental health. This important book adds a clinically informed and clearly articulated set of tools and insights to the discussion of how we shall adapt to an ecologically changing world. This resource for resilience puts psychotherapeutic tools and ecological science in service to personal and social wellbeing."

—*Craig Chalquist, Department Chair East-West Psychology at California Institute of Integral Studies and author of* Terrapsychology: Reengaging the Soul of Place

"Leslie's work marks a much-needed advancement for the integration of mental health and broader context of climate change and environmental threats. She goes further than recognizing the importance of this connection, however—she provides a framework and methodology for supporting those on the front lines of the mental health professions. I know this work will be valued and appreciated by many, and will ultimately support all of our collective efforts to repair and mend our world."

—*Renee Lertzman, author of* Environmental Melancholia

"*Emotional Resiliency for the Era of Climate Change* is a courageous exploration of the impact that facing the realities of climate change can have on people's mental health and well-being, and a much-needed catalyst for teaching people tools of resiliency in a time of planet-wide crisis. The author is bold in her vision, both evocative and encouraging, and skillful in teaching the reflections and exercises that guide the reader from grief, confusion, or passivity through needed shifts in perspectives and lifestyle to wise, grounded, effective action."

—*Linda Graham, author of* Bouncing Back: Rewiring Your
Brain for Maximum Resilience and Well-Being

"This comprehensive and compassionate gem of a book, with its wealth of practical wisdom and transformational practices, is exactly what the helping professions (and all of us) need to be of service to one another in the face of the ongoing ecological trauma that is our most urgent global challenge."

—*Miriam Greenspan, author of* Healing through the Dark Emotions

"Leslie Davenport has written an important guide to help all of us with the psychological challenges associated with climate change. This book not only provides the reader with a concise summary of how Earth's climate is changing, but more importantly, it provides compassionate, practical guidance on ways to deal with the dis-ease surrounding this issue. Therapists, clients and the general public will all benefit from the wisdom this book holds regarding civilizations greatest challenge: human caused climate change."

—*Jeffrey T. Kiehl, Jungian Analyst, author of* Facing Climate
Change: An Integrated Path to the Future

"*Emotional Resiliency in the Era of Climate Change* is a pioneering, time-sensitive book that is a must-read right now in order to prepare, heal, and transform our human inter-relationship with climate change. Davenport has written an intellectually wise and heartfelt book that provides scientific and practical exercises to move through climate change denial, access resilience, and unleash both personal and planetary healing.

While this book primarily calls forth on mental health professionals to embrace climate change as an essential aspect of assessment and treatment, this book is also the extremely valuable for anyone interested in fostering increased self-care, embodied wisdom, and compassionate living in relation to the natural world. The worksheets in Part I combined with the 12 exercises are also extremely beneficial for educators, activists, first responders, and other helping citizens."

—*Laury Rappaport, Founder and Director of Focusing and Expressive Arts
Institute, author of* Mindfulness and the Arts Therapies: Theory and Practice

"In this very readable book, Leslie Davenport offers profound insights into the psychological causes of climate change denial (which we all suffer from to some extent), suggestions about how we can break through it with courage, integrity, and resiliency, and powerful practices to help. Although it is written especially for therapists, this book is for everyone, because we all face the catastrophic effects of climate change."

—*Molly Brown, co-author with Joanna Macy of* Coming Back to
Life: The Updated Guide to the Work that Reconnects

Emotional
Resiliency
in the Era of
Climate Change

by the same author

Transformative Imagery
Cultivating the Imagination for Healing, Change, and Growth
Edited by Leslie Davenport
Foreword by Martin L. Rossman
ISBN 978 1 84905 742 4
eISBN 978 1 78450 175 4

of related interest

With Nature in Mind
The Ecotherapy Manual for Mental Health Professionals
Andy McGeeney
Foreword by Lindsay Royan
ISBN 978 1 78592 024 0
eISBN 978 1 78450 270 6

Emotional Resiliency in the Era of Climate Change

A Clinician's Guide

Leslie Davenport

Foreword by Lise Van Susteren, M.D.

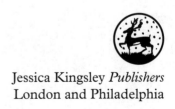

Jessica Kingsley *Publishers*
London and Philadelphia

The photo on p.92 is courtesy of Ignacio Jarero, Ph.D., senior EMDR trainer and founder of Amamecrisis, Mexico. The photo on p.102 is courtesy of Center for Council: www.centerforcouncil.org

First published in 2017
by Jessica Kingsley Publishers
73 Collier Street
London N1 9BE, UK
and
400 Market Street, Suite 400
Philadelphia, PA 19106, USA

www.jkp.com

Copyright © Leslie Davenport 2017
Foreword copyright © Lise Van Susteren 2017

Front cover image source: Stocksnap.io

Library of Congress Cataloging in Publication Data
A CIP catalog record for this book is available from the Library of Congress

British Library Cataloguing in Publication Data
A CIP catalogue record for this book is available from the British Library

ISBN 978 1 78592 719 5
eISBN 978 1 78450 328 4

Printed and bound in the United States

For my children's children.
May wild grace guide our actions
that all beings may thrive.

Contents

FOREWORD

We have been warned repeatedly, and with a deepening sense of anguish, by scientists from every corner of the world that the impacts of climate change on civilization and the natural world are accelerating. Our planet is on fire. We have daily news of floods, droughts, wildfires, and a cascade of extreme weather events claiming lives, property, and community. But it isn't just the physical toll all this is having on us, it is also, increasingly, the psychological toll. As climate-change-induced anxiety, trauma, and depression broaden and deepen, in the years to come meeting the mental health needs of humanity will be a critical and central challenge.

Mental health professionals are uniquely qualified to address these issues as well as the problematic behaviors that cause them. We help people see how denial and resistance to change can mean worse trouble down the road for themselves, their families, their communities. We help people face reality and in doing so promote the kinds of choices that build emotional resilience and move us towards positive change. We are good at offering effective ways to communicate to facilitate both personal and systemic changes. Aren't we, as mental health professionals, just the right people to be at the epicenter of the battle to save our home from climate change? Where then, we have to ask, are all our colleagues and the institutional support that would help the world address this unprecedented crisis?

We are in the midst of climate-linked water wars, civil wars, food insecurity, national insecurity, diminished biodiversity, and the rise of displacement, diseases, and violence. Though as mental health professionals we are in the swirl of many directions, our professional mission statements mandate that we make a commitment to relieve human suffering. It is hard to imagine a more compelling cause than taking action to address the suffering from the impacts of climate change.

Activism is tough work. Many of the most dedicated "warriors" are deeply worried, some are burned out, all suffer from a frantic sadness they seek to alleviate with their efforts to awaken the world to action. Many struggle with a post-traumatic stress disorder (PTSD) like syndrome—a "pre-traumatic stress disorder" that has them relentlessly envisioning future harm.

Leslie Davenport has taken a much-needed next step that brings together psychology's best practices with the specific mental health needs of people suffering from the impacts of climate change. Her book acknowledges the harsh realities of our changing world and offers a comprehensive collection of heartfelt tools for encouraging effective action and emotional resilience. It is a book about positive change—both inner and outer—in a unified direction that will support us in transforming ourselves and bringing our relationship with the natural world into a life-sustaining balance.

We know it's no longer enough simply to unleash more startling facts and blast images of our planet being violated. We also need to cultivate a pragmatic form of hope by helping develop empowering actions, a clear direction, ways to connect with collective and systemic support, practices for effective self-care, and the tools and methods necessary for change. By taking a dive into the prospects and practices that this book offers, we will all learn to do just that.

The book is an invitation to personal and professional transformation—one that strengthens our integrity and prepares us for action. Leslie expands the role of mental health practitioners, showing how professional development can prepare our field for engaging in this work. Seasoned professionals will find valuable ways to discover unexamined biases, resolve personal insecurities, and activate untapped resources. Essential methodologies are distilled into worksheets that can be made available to clients for fostering new insights and strengthening capabilities.

The emotional intelligence required to respond fully to climate change demands a deepening awareness that we are a part of nature and that nature is a part of us. Our interconnectedness is more apparent and vital than ever, and so is the need to engage. And going beyond personal fulfillment, it is our collective effort that is needed for the urgent social and political evolution our planet's condition requires.

We must act now, charting a course of ecoharmony together…linked by common purpose and determination. *Emotional Resiliency in the Era of Climate Change* provides what we need for the journey ahead.

Lise Van Susteren, M.D.
Washington DC
July 16, 2016

ACKNOWLEDGMENTS

For most of my life I have been exploring how we can thrive throughout the full gamut of life's dangers and joys, actualizing our unique expressions while living in harmony with our wildly diverse animal and human family. My intention for this book is to provide both the inspiration and the tools to map this trajectory of growth, offering what I've discovered. My heartfelt thanks go to Jessica Kingsley Publishers for sharing this vision; they consistently publish books that make a difference. Their staff has been a joy to work with.

While this book ventures into new psychological territory, it is built on the foundation of my lifelong work. During my 25-year career in the medical world, I worked to create a collaborative model for resolving crisis and empowering healing, and this has influenced my approach to climate psychology. Most recently, my experiences at COP21 in Paris and my participation in 350.org and the Pachamama Alliance have given momentum to this book.

My gratitude also goes to all those who shared themselves so generously. Deep respect and appreciation go to my editor, Madeleine Fahrenwald, who understands what I am trying to say, sometimes even between the lines, and has a way of helping me express the message even more clearly. Special thanks to Mark Spain, Juanita De Sanz, and Laury Rappaport who read a draft and offered their insights and wisdom. A late-night conversation with Nancy Dunn helped bring focus to some key themes. I hope to have many more of those fun, no-nonsense dialogues with her. Elizabeth Baker, Jade Wood, and Nichole Warwick connected me with people who provided contributions during the formation of this book, and Nina Simons took time from her intense schedule for a consultation. Gaybriella Igno rescued me from technical brambles when I was designing the visual diagrams and preparing photos that illustrate the book.

Warm appreciation to Lori Cheek and to many in the community of Jamestown, Colorado, about whom you will be reading in these pages. They were so willing to openly share their intimate and inspiring stories of resiliency; their invitation to witness and learn from their paths is a service to us all.

I feel loving gratitude for my family, friends, colleagues, and clients for supporting and shaping me in the most powerful and surprising ways, as I continue to discover ways of exploring and serving the harsh and beautiful quandaries of life.

Introduction

We find ourselves at a pivotal time in human history, an era marked by heightened peril and tremendous possibility. Climate change is bringing humanity to a crisis point (Knieling and Filho 2012), with some scientists warning that if we continue on our current trajectory we will create a planetary environment inhospitable to life (Fyall 2009). Yet in the midst of this dark, painful time there is a surprising gift available, a radical invitation to a profound transformation. We can aim to go beyond protecting the environment to creating the kind of world where the environment is no longer in need of protecting.

I invite you to…

…embrace a vision—backed by action—of clean air and water for our children and our children's children

…incline your heart and mind more frequently toward the realization of our interdependent relationship with all of life

…build a future where we can enjoy and respect a rich diversity of plants, animals, and people that are thriving on our planet

…recognize that what we do now will either enhance or degrade the future lent us by our children.

Addressing climate change is more than reducing carbon emissions and creating clean-energy solutions. Tackling the practical aspects of a sustainable future is a vital part of our evolution—but taking a deeper look is crucial. At this juncture we are compelled to examine the beliefs and values that propelled us to this tipping point. If we can recognize the vital connection between our thoughts, emotions, and behavior in our moment-to-moment choices, the damaging costs to people and the environment can be eliminated. This shift empowers a new way of seeing that can guide us to develop a conscious and responsible relationship to the whole, of which we are but a part.

Many perennial philosophies, as well as modern-day systems theory, have described the interdependence of all things, life as a web-like system where one action influences all others (Thiele 2013), and Interbeing (Hạnh 1987), where all of life—human and non-human elements—are interconnected and contained within the other.

> If you are a poet, you will see clearly that there is a cloud floating in this sheet of paper. Without a cloud, there will be no rain; without rain, the trees cannot grow; and without trees, we cannot make paper. The cloud is essential for the paper to exist. If the cloud is not here, the sheet of paper cannot be here either. So we can say that the cloud and the paper inter-are. "Interbeing" is a word that is not in the dictionary yet, but if we combine the prefix "inter-" with the verb "to be," we have a new verb, inter-be. (Hạnh and Ellsberg 2001, p.55)

Now we are directly experiencing what this actually means in practical terms, which holds great hope for building our understanding of what is required for sustainable life. We can now directly observe the impact between our deep, often unexamined beliefs and climate change. Our Western lifestyle is dangerously disconnected from a true understanding of interdependence.

In the simplest terms, our awareness (or lack thereof) shapes our beliefs, which in turn instruct our lifestyle. In developed nations in particular, our way of life requires burning enormous amounts of fossil fuels that emit greenhouses gases. These emissions get trapped as heat in the atmosphere, causing the earth to warm. The increasing temperature changes climate patterns and, depending on the area, creates drought, floods, and intensified storms. Ice is melting at the poles, threatening an extreme rise in sea levels that is already impacting coastal areas.

The oceans are warming, killing krill and reefs essential to the sea-based food supply chain. The increased heat is triggering the extinctions of species where plants and animals are unable to adapt quickly enough to their rapidly changing environment. Food and water supplies are becoming depleted, which impacts all types of communities and amplifies economic security issues as we compete more and more for our basic life needs. Air and water pollution are contributing to health problems, especially among the most vulnerable populations, including children, the elderly, and underserved regions (Field *et al.* 2012).

While burning fossil fuels has been a key factor in the escalation of global warming, the root causes of the current damage to the earth—and ultimately ourselves—are more complex and multidimensional. Much of our industrialized society contains insidious systems that are unsustainable and produce measurable harm. Nocuous practices can be found within the agro-food business, a high-consumption lifestyle designed for single-use, disposable plastic items and short-lived, high-tech devices, supported by a widespread disregard for working conditions and fair-trade values and all fueled by deceptive advertising driven by corporate and political forces that reject transparency and accountability.

As we dive more deeply into the facts about how climate change is damaging all forms of life on the earth, it is truly frightening. There may be times when facing the truth just feels too bewildering, too hard. Reading this book and engaging in this work require emotional buoyancy—but know that it's a process where feelings naturally ebb and flow. If we are lucky, we can maintain a humble attitude of learning. We can challenge ourselves to continue building skill, depth of heart, and clear seeing, and then keep showing up. We can summon the courage to open to the human experience of our current era and find our humanity—grieve the pain and engage in hopeful actions in tandem with our clients. We can reach out and connect heart-to-heart with others who are doing this work too.

In this book, you will find resiliency tools alongside the climate science described, so that you can build internal strength and help find solutions as we join the most important work of our time. These chapters will reveal the status of the climate change chaos on our planet, but know that they'll also present creative and effective technologies and lifestyles that can serve as excellent models for both action and healing. I invite you now to take a breath. Commend yourself for entering this work as a compassionate and peaceful warrior, as we move on to learn more about the psychological impacts of climate change.

As devastating as the losses of resources, species, security, health, and property are, we have yet to awaken fully to the psychological suffering that is inextricably linked to these changes. We do not have to look far to find examples of communities struggling to cope with the psychological impact of environmental disasters. In neighborhoods affected by Hurricane Katrina, 39 percent experienced moderate post-traumatic stress disorder symptoms and 24 percent had severe symptoms. Suicide attempts were 78.6 times higher than the area's baseline rate. There was also an increase in depression and domestic violence (Balaban *et al.* 2012, pp.9–11).

Similar emotional trauma was found among the evacuees of the Fukushima nuclear disaster. Close to a year after Japan's earthquake, tsunami, and nuclear crisis, the National Institute of Mental Health in Tokyo assessed 91,000 people and discovered that the experience of extreme stress was five times the normal rate, with one in five individuals exhibiting symptoms of trauma. In children, the stress levels were double the national average (Brumfiel 2013, p.6).

As I write this book, the United States is relocating its first climate refugees. Isle de Jean Charles, Louisiana is sinking into the sea, and families who have lived there for generations have been forced to leave. Federal monies were allocated to relocate an entire community, primarily tribal residents of the Biloxi-Chitimacha-Choctaw and United Houma Nation. It is not only about mildewed homes and fruit trees dying from salt water in the soil; Chief Albert Naquin also mourns, "We're going to lose all our heritage, all our culture" (Davenport and Robertson 2016, p.1).

Climate scientists predict that natural disasters will be harsher and more frequent than we have ever experienced before (Finneran 2013). Along with these devastating events, the Executive Summary of the *Psychological Effects of Global Warming on the United States* warns that, "Global warming...in the coming years...will foster public trauma, depression, violence, alienation, substance abuse, suicide, psychotic episodes, post-traumatic stress disorders and many other mental health-related conditions" (Balaban *et al.* 2012, p.i). The numbers impacted are staggering: it is estimated that in the coming years, 200 million Americans will be touched by significant psychological distress from climate-related events (Balaban *et al.* 2012, p.v). Many other parts of the world will continue to have more concentrated and profound exposure to loss and even fewer resources to address the devastation (Marshall *et al.* 2012).

How can we find our way through this frightening time? Where is the potential for transformation, and how can we engage in it?

While the process is multifaceted and non-linear, we first need to be willing to see clearly what is occurring and face the pain of our current global distress. Not surprisingly, the forward-looking climate scientists who have been mapping out potential scenarios are now using phrases like "climate depression" (Thomas 2014) and "pre-traumatic stress" (Holmes 2015) to describe their own overwhelming fear, anger, and sadness mixed with a profound uncertainty about what the future may hold. Camille Parmesan, a lead author of the *Third Assessment Report* from the Intergovernmental Panel on Climate Change winner of the Nobel Peace Prize, affirms this, "I do not know of a single scientist that is not having an emotional reaction to what is being lost" (Thomas 2014, p.2). It naturally follows that as the findings are more extensively read, and the climate impacts more widely felt, the psychological distress will also increase proportionately.

There is good reason to grieve the state of life on our planet, and allowing the experience of grief is part of the healing. When we mourn, it gradually clears a path that frees up our emotional energy so that it can be used to pursue new possibilities and take positive action.

While grief is painful, the process also contains a powerful transformative component. As we face losses, whether they are aspects of our lifestyle, resources, or even a shifting sense of self, grief is preparing the soil of our psyche. It is uprooting olds beliefs and loosening our internal ground, which has been tamped down by habit and routine. Potential is uncovered. The process moves toward an invitation to reexamine ourselves and our relationship to life, planting new seeds of possibility in our fertile hearts and minds. This understanding of grief and transformation has been examined for centuries. The 13th-century Persian poet Rumi said it this way:

> Sorrow prepares you for joy. It violently sweeps everything out of your house, so that new joy can find space to enter. It shakes the yellow leaves from the bough of your heart, so that fresh, green leaves can grow in their place. It pulls up the rotten roots, so that new roots hidden beneath have room to grow. Whatever sorrow shakes from your heart, far better things will take their place (Bill and Chavez 2002, p.575).

The role of climate change psychology

Mental health practitioners have an invaluable role to play at this pivotal time in history. An article in *American Psychologist* goes so far as to assert that, "Psychologists have an ethical obligation to take immediate steps to minimize the psychological harm associated with climate change, to help to reduce global disparities in climate impacts, and to continually improve their climate-related interventions through coordinated programs of research and practice that draw on the rich diversity of psychologists' skills and training" (Doherty and Clayton 2011, p.273).

This book presents a broad understanding of climate change as a context for delving more deeply into the psychosocial interfaces. The process of building resilience, both for ourselves and as psychotherapists for our clients, is approached at four levels of climate change psychology.

1. CLIMATE CONVERSATIONS THAT REACH THROUGH DENIAL

The book examines the many reasons why it is difficult for people to recognize, and even talk about, our changing environment. Recommendations are offered for effective ways to engage in dialogues that dig deep into our collective distress and take action instead of floating in paralysis or denial.

2. CHRONIC, LOW-LEVEL STRESS

As people become more aware of what is actually occurring on our warming planet, anxiety, grief, and helplessness can take hold. The book includes the most successful ways to build confidence and hope while addressing the full range of thoughts and feelings.

3. ACUTE, HIGH-IMPACT TRAUMA

With the intensification and frequency of climate-change-induced disasters—hurricanes, drought-related fires, floods—more mental health professions are needed to respond effectively to disaster trauma. An updated model of disaster response that incorporates mindfulness is presented.

4. Restorative/transformational model

Mental health professionals also have valuable tools for ushering forth powerful transitions in consciousness and behavior that can lead to sustainable lifestyles that foster a healthy humanity and planet. This transition can ultimately lead to a reimagining of the world where true community engagement is practiced, contentment is valued over consumption, respect for the full impact of daily choices is transparently lived, gratitude accompanies everyday moments, and the grandeur of the natural world engenders a sense of awe.

Deep resilience

Resilience is a process of skillfully navigating through crisis with the ability to psychologically "bounce back" from times of high distress. With climate change, the challenges are large in scale, long-term, and complex, and we need to enhance our capacities and reach deep for our most sustaining connections within ourselves and one another.

Resilience can be learned by virtually anyone, and there are deep resiliency practices and perspectives woven throughout the chapters of this book. The more the practices are engaged, the stronger and more available these resources become. A few of the many features of resiliency include accepting the reality of change, focusing on what can be done, engaging in meaningful conversations and action, nurturing creativity, encouraging flexibility and curiosity, expanding mindful awareness of the connections between thoughts, emotions, physiology, and joining with others to build community. We have the freedom to choose to live by our most sovereign values.

Models for working with trauma, anxiety, and grief are well established in psychotherapeutic theory and practice, but there are no clear clinical guidelines or paradigms that address the overarching psychological effects of climate change. The mental health system as a whole is underprepared to handle the magnitude of the stressors on the horizon (Balaban *et al.* 2012). This book offers strategies and resources for mental health clinicians, and portions of the book will also be useful for first responders, healthcare professionals, life coaches, and community disaster-response volunteers.

Emotional Resiliency in the Era of Climate Change synthesizes core clinical themes and evidence-based best practices drawn from expert clinical research in areas including ecopsychology, disaster-response training, trauma, and grief work, as well as transformative resilience practices from positive psychology, wisdom traditions, mindfulness teachings, creative therapies, "intentional community" circles, earth-based indigenous practices, and guided imagery.

How to use this book

Reading the entire book provides an in-depth understanding of the issues involved and treatment options to address the psychospiritual effects of climate change. The chapters can also be used as stand-alone references when specific concerns arise with a client or population. The worksheets found at the end of each chapter in Part I are available to download from www.jkp.com/voucher using the code DAVENPORTCLIMATE. The book is in two sections:

PART I: CLINICAL THEMES IN THE ERA OF CLIMATE CHANGE

Each chapter has three components:

1. A clinical understanding of the presenting issue with treatment recommendations.

2. A worksheet that lists therapeutic practices that can be copied and provided to clients or groups.

3. Additional resources for extended study of the topic.

Chapter 1: The Psychology of Climate Change Denial
WORKSHEET: CLARITY AND SELF-CARE
Why do people turn away from the realities of climate change? This chapter answers this question and introduces processes that help us talk about and come to terms with the current state of the planet. In order to do this work, clinicians must also commit to and practice self-care in order to attend to their own experience of loss and to prevent professional burnout. The first worksheet is recommended for both mental health practitioners and clients.

Chapter 2: Climate Change Grief
WORKSHEET: MAPPING YOUR GRIEF JOURNEY
AND EXPLORING PRIVILEGE

An emerging model of the stages of climate grief (Running 2007) is presented. Guidelines and practices are provided that increase our tolerance for and ultimately honor the complex array of feelings unique to our time and that help us convert emotional pain into transformative action. The distinction between empathy and compassion is explored. With climate grief in particular, attitude and behavior are intimately connected, and both must be transformed in order to achieve a full resolution.

Chapter 3: An Overview of Clinical Themes Involving Climate Change
WORKSHEET: TRANSFORMATIONAL LEADERSHIP

This chapter introduces the broad spectrum of clinical issues that can be triggered by a climate change event, using a case study. It also reveals the ways that resiliency can spontaneously arise and be fostered in the therapeutic recovery process. This chapter describes how mental health professionals can take a leadership role to support regenerative transformation, both individually and culturally.

Chapter 4: Mindful Disaster Response: Perspectives from Ground Zero
WORKSHEET: RESILIENCY PRACTICES

Interventions that are the most effective in mitigating the psychological impact of climate-change-induced catastrophes are explored, including "therapy without walls" at the disaster site. The upheavals of intense emotion that manifest in conjunction with multiple losses, underlying mental health issues, and collective trauma will be explained, and guidelines are offered for assessing the level of psychological mediation required in the various stages of recovery. Research and practices on the effectiveness of mindfulness in trauma recovery are provided.

Chapter 5: Long-term and Complex Clinical Themes
WORKSHEET: MORAL INJURY—FORGIVING
OURSELVES, FORGIVING OTHERS

As we endeavor to talk about new climate-induced experiences and the deep feelings that accompany them, creative language is emerging.

Solastalgia, a new psychological term that refers to environment-induced stress (Weissbecker 2011), will be explored along with the themes of vicarious traumatization, survivor guilt, recovery fatigue, moral injury, and coping with increased diseases. Empowerment strategies include self-compassion, healthy boundaries, and forgiveness practices. Evidence-based mind–body tools that can promote emotional resiliency and support health and wellbeing are also included.

Chapter 6: Resiliency Stories
WORKSHEET: LISTENING TO YOUR HEART
AND THE HEART OF THE EARTH

Climate change psychology is an endeavor of hope. This chapter illustrates several examples of more awakened and resilient living that is rising from the ashes and mud in areas that are experiencing climate distress. It also looks at ecovillages, intentional communities with a proactive and green design. A transformation is already in the making, and this chapter highlights examples of the creative momentum that we can join and encourage.

PART II: VITALIZATION OF AN ECOHARMONIOUS LIFE: TWELVE BODY, HEART/MIND, AND WORLD WISE PRACTICES

One of the most useful tools for activating an ecoharmonious life is our imagination. As we create radically new visions of our relationship to the earth and our culture, our imaginations illuminate further creative possibilities. This section contains 12 practices that will help reconnect with our original nature, tap into our creative wisdom, and integrate our way of being in the world with a heightened experience of interdependence with nature in order to reshape our relationship with the world. I recommend that you to use a journal to dive deeply into the practices. It is beneficial to write out the questions posed in each practice and record your reflections with free-form writing, action commitments, drawings, or even collages. Allow plenty of space for each practice, so that you can return to them and add related quotes and inspirations from a range of sources, deepening and expanding the themes over time. Blending your creative, visionary perspectives with practical action steps will encourage grounded transformation.

There are three parts to each practice.

- **Body Wise** begins each practice with simple movements, postures, or stretches, often including breathing exercises that promote self-care, reduce stress, increase physical wellbeing and somatic awareness, and help us listen to the wisdom of the body.

- **Heart/Mind Wise** brings kind attention to stressful emotions like worry, anger, and regret. Tools for experiencing the full range of feelings are introduced as we move toward emotional resiliency, learning to shift our focus to the wisdom arising from a clear mind and open heart.

- **World Wise** opens the door to experiencing the wonder, awe, and mystery of life in simple everyday moments. These practices provide a healthy structure for grounding our insights and intention into action and connecting with others and the world.

The transformative journey has already begun and we are part of it. Each day, the life story is unfolding through everyone's decisions, lifestyles, and ways of being. Because we are not separate from nature and all of life, our hearts, minds, and talents are part of the remedy. As therapists we can utilize our training to help others plumb the depths of their hearts, grieve the pain of our era, and transfigure their lives with an ecoharmonious connection at the center. This is meaningful work and a formidable responsibility.

Unfortunately, our profession does not exempt us from the direct impacts of climate change on our own lives. It is likely that your own heart will break open many times in this work. Those cracks can also usher forth sacred creativity and rewild your heart, letting in the astounding beauty of life. This book will help you and your clients convert climate change suffering into a fuel for transformation.

In those times when it feels like we are struggling to keep our own heart above water, remember that the world needs each one of us. Systems theorist Buckminster Fuller reminds us:

Never forget that you are one of a kind. Never forget that if there weren't any need for you in all your uniqueness to be on this earth, you wouldn't be here in the first place. And never forget, no matter how overwhelming life's challenges and problems seem to be, that one person can make a difference in the world. In fact, it is always because of one person that all the changes that matter in the world come about. So be that one person. (Petras and Petras 2009, p.97)

We are not in this alone. People are rising up to assume shared responsibility for a collective and systemic approach. There are scientists, artists, engineers, farmers, clergy, students, celebrities, parents, activists, and world leaders who are also committed to finding their way toward lifestyles and professions that are ecoharmonious while working to halt and repair the damage inflicted upon ourselves and the living earth. This kind of participation requires that we discern clarity about our part in the transformative process; enliven our intention and commitment without perfectionism; and become fully involved in a balanced way that encourages self-care and even joy.

Lise Van Susteren, a psychiatrist and advisor with the Harvard Medical School Center for Health and the Global Environment, makes a passionate plea:

Mental health professionals vigorously endorse requirements to report cases of child abuse. It is a legal obligation, but it is also a moral one. Is it any less compelling a moral obligation, in the name of all children now and in the future, to report that we are on track to hand over a planet that may be destroyed for generations to come? I respectfully request that we, as mental health professionals, make a unified stand in support of actions to reduce the threat of catastrophic climate change. (Van Susteren 2011, p.1)

Will you join us?

Additional resources

Intergovernmental Panel on Climate Change: www.ipcc.ch (a leading international body of researchers on climate change, established by the United Nations).

Jung, C. G. (2002) *The Earth Has a Soul: C.G. Jung on Nature, Technology, and Modern Life.* Berkeley, CA: North Atlantic Books.

Macy, J. and Brown, M. (2014) *Coming Back to Life: The Updated Guide to the Work that Reconnects.* Gabriola Island, BC, Canada: New Society Publishers.

Swim, J., Clayton, S., Doherty, T., Gifford, R. *et al.* (2009) *Psychology and Global Climate Change: Addressing a Multifaceted Phenomenon and Set of Challenges.* Washington, DC: American Psychological Association. Available at: www.apa. org/science/about/publications/climate-change-booklet.pdf, accessed on 19 August 2016.

Part I

Clinical Themes in the Era of Climate Change

Chapter 1

The Psychology of Climate Change Denial

Awakening to the severity of climate change happens to us in many ways. For some it is subtle: we detect confusing shifts in the natural world, such as delicate spring flowers blossoming in winter, or we have to cancel our annual ski trip due to lack of snow. Initially, it is easy to find these kinds of events surprising without necessarily feeling alarmed. As we notice more shifts in the natural rhythms of nature, we begin to have a growing sense of something wrong, a quiet but fundamental unease. Perhaps these unsettling feelings are amplified by an evening news report on record temperatures, like the winter of 2015, when one temperature recorded at the North Pole hit 50 degrees above normal (Samenow 2015). For others, the truth of climate disruption rushes in dramatically when coastal waters unexpectedly submerge their family home. In whatever ways we hear nature's distressed voice, whether it is gradual or sudden, what often follows is a flood of feelings that can include fear, powerlessness, overwhelm, grief, and despair.

Since climate change has been called one of the greatest threats facing life on the planet, and more and more people are directly affected by its disruptions, why does there continue to be a lack of sufficient engagement with this topic? It is logical that a growing body of scientific information and the increasing number of climate disasters would spur individuals, governments, and corporations to take meaningful action—but this is generally not the case. When we look at both our deeply programmed stress reactions and motivational studies, it becomes clear why climate change denial is so strongly entrenched.

Current beliefs about climate change in the United States

In March 2015, the Yale Project on Climate Change Communication and the George Mason University Center for Climate Communication released a survey of 1,200 adults' attitudes and beliefs about climate change in the United States. Here are a few of the key findings.

BELIEFS AND ATTITUDES

- Three in ten (32%) say they believe global warming is due mostly to natural changes in the environment. About half of Americans (52%) think that global warming, if they believe it is actually happening, is mostly human-caused. That number jumped to 65 percent in 2016, according to a Gallup Poll (Saad and Jones 2016).

- Only about one in ten Americans understand that over 90 percent of climate scientists think human-caused global warming is occurring.

- About half of Americans (52%) say they are at least "somewhat worried" about global warming, but only 11 percent say they are "very worried" about it.

- Only about one in three Americans (32%) think people in the United States are being harmed "right now" by global warming.

COMMUNICATION

- Most Americans (74%) say they "rarely" or "never" discuss global warming with family and friends, a number that has grown substantially since 2008 (60%).

Policy support

- About one in four Americans (26%) are currently part of—or would "definitely" or "probably" be willing to join—a campaign to convince elected officials to take action to reduce global warming (Leiserowitz *et al.* 2015, pp.3–4).

So perhaps this survey suggests that we need more climate change facts disseminated to the public more quickly. While improved media coverage would be beneficial, the psychology of change reveals that this would not be a full solution.

Bill McKibben—author, activist, and the man the *Boston Globe* called "probably America's most important environmentalist" (Mandel 2015, p.1)—reveals his own learning curve on communicating about the state of the environment. When his book *The End of Nature* was released in 1989, it was a bestseller that was translated into several dozen languages. He states simply, "My initial theory…was that people would read the book—and then change" (McKibben 2013, p.7). He goes on to describe spending years pursuing the same approach: more books, more articles, more lectures. But it was precisely the lack of meaningful response that resulted from his efforts, including from those who remained complacent after exposure to the hard science, that led him to become a self-described "unlikely activist" (McKibben 2013, front cover) and to search for different and more effective ways to engage others with his message. This resulted in his creation of 350.org, a "global grassroots climate movement that can hold our leaders accountable to the realities of science and the principles of justice," that is active in over 188 countries (350.org 2016, homepage).

Psychology has long confirmed that people do not change their behavior based on data (Heath and Heath 2010). This is easily recognized in the domain of health psychology's strategies for lifestyle change, such as stop-smoking and nutrition campaigns. Simply providing a wealth of information on the cancer-causing, disease-producing impacts of unhealthy habits rarely leads to the desired outcome. Instead, many factors for promoting a healthy shift need to complement the educational component, including focusing on the specific benefits of healthy choices, peer and professional support, practical tools for shifting deeply ingrained habits, and, most importantly, ways to address and process emotional responses and examine beliefs and assumptions that often dwell just below our conscious awareness. Without the deeper work, our underlying psychological foundation remains more powerful than the facts, blocking the most urgently needed responses and preventing engagement. This is definitely true when it comes to the lifestyle and policy changes required to impact climate change.

There are also some specific climate-related features that interface with our psychological makeup detailed through the chapter that reinforce our denial. As we diagnose the sources of resistance, they will provide the keys to effective change—individually and in the larger system.

Climate disruption and stress responses: fight, flight, and freeze

The familiar trio of adaptive stress responses that are hardwired into our body's survival repertoire can be a useful lens for examining our reactions to climate-related threats. They are completely natural and deeply engrained responses to danger. While individuals have a primary tendency toward one of the three primitive reactions, we are fluid: we move between fight (when we believe we have the potential to defeat the threat), flight (if the force is too powerful, our impulse is to escape), and freeze (when we can neither defend ourselves nor outrun the danger). The three physiological reactions evolved for brief, immediate threats, but these reactive states are prolonged in modern-day life and have been shown to erode our physical health and contribute to emotional depletion. As our stress reactions also manifest in response to climate distress, they not only have adverse effects on the individual, they even sabotage our opportunity to create much-needed change.

The upcoming examples of stress responses to climate issues require our discernment: we need real commitment to the climate movement in order to reverse our current destructive path, but rigid engagement can become obsessional and harden into an unintended obstacle. We need self-care, but when we seek balance it can be easy to slide into distancing and avoidance.

Discernment can be subtle. The "fight" response described below is *not* imputed to all individuals who have an abiding commitment to environmental work and place it at the center of their lives. It also does not refer to the healthy outrage that surfaces when we respond to the magnitude of destruction that is presently occurring. Nor does it describe all those who take a stand and push back or "fight" against injustice in some way. There is a valuable seed in each of the examples, but you will see how the core benefits of activism can coalesce into a counterproductive shadow dynamic when we are primarily fueled by stress. There are subtle but distinct qualitative differences between those who have developed a clear and grounded approach to climate work and those who are primarily acting out stress reactions.

CLIMATE PSYCHOLOGY AND THE STRESS REACTION: FIGHT

The "fight" stress reaction is characterized by those who have a knee-jerk reaction to "come out swinging" when faced with a stressful situation. Some individuals in this reactive state jump into extreme activism. This can show up as excessive activity, reckless language, argumentativeness, and impulsive, obsessive, and addictive behaviors. Their personal lives may be out of balance. Those who react in this way to their distress about climate change can spend hours blasting social media posts, blogging, and news-bingeing. In some cases, their activity can even escalate into violent action. Climate advocates operating in this mode seem to believe that if they shout the information louder and more frequently, it will force things to shift (and psychoanalytically speaking, reduce their own stress). But as Deborah Tannen, Professor of Linguistics at Georgetown University clarifies, "Smashing heads does not open minds" (Tannen 1999, p.26).

Paradoxical environmental numbness

Many environmental activists of this type genuinely hope to spur others into taking action, but they do not recognize the limitations of their approach. Robert Gifford, Professor of Psychology and Environmental Studies at the University of Victoria (British Columbia, Canada), paints a picture of what the outcome can be when others are exposed to this kind of activism. He reports that when people are given a great deal of information about the environmental dangers of climate chaos without having had a direct experience of personal difficulties related to it, they tend to tune out after a while, creating a kind of "environmental numbness" (Gifford, Kormos, and McIntyre 2011). According to Per Espen Stoknes of the Center for Climate Strategies in Norway, religious groups that focus on social justice can experience the same phenomenon, framed in those circles as "apocalypse fatigue" (Stoknes 2014). Strategies that arouse regret or fear were confirmed as the least effective for encouraging change in 129 different behavior-change studies (Curfman 2009). These results are clear examples of how well-intended but out-of-balance efforts can produce the opposite of the desired effects.

Solution aversion

Some environmental activists caught in the fight response also become solution-averse, using hot-button phrases that can close down conversations rather than initiating valuable dialogue. They will often split the world (and even other environmental groups) into good and bad, a black-and-white style of thinking that leads to infighting and division rather than collaboration. This is also known as the "extremist effect," and it is characterized by rigidity, demonizing others, and control. Dr. Amy Gutmann, Professor in the Annenberg School for Communication at the University of Pennsylvania, describes two defining features of extremist rhetoric: it tends toward single-mindedness and "passionately expresses certainty about the supremacy of its perspective" (Gutmann 2007, p.1).

These activists' messages may be largely true and their passion fueled by a reasonable sense of urgency. But studies of interpersonal and organizational communication repeatedly reveal that *how* ideas are communicated is as much or more important than *what* is expressed, in terms of gaining the desired result. We know there are large groups of people interested in learning more about climate action and making changes, but they struggle against strongly held personal beliefs. When these groups are on the receiving end of blame or judgment from "fighters" and are vilified for not acting quickly enough—or they feel assaulted by rigidly held views of how they should be living—these groups are alienated rather than helped to move through the questions and feelings that would enable them to join the movement (Campbell and Kay 2014). These "fighter" activists also have a high risk of burnout.

CLIMATE PSYCHOLOGY AND THE STRESS REACTION: FLIGHT

Susan Clayton, a psychology professor and Chair of the Environmental Studies program at the College of Wooster in Ohio, captures the essence of the "flight" reaction when she remarks, "In a way, it's kind of surprising that anybody pays attention... We don't want to think about something that's scary" (Roewe 2015, p.1). This is understandable:

we want to avoid pain, especially when it appears that there is no clear solution. When we learn of a potential threat, it is natural and also anxiety-provoking to wonder, "Where can I go to be safe? What's going to happen to me and the people, places, and things I love and care about?"

We humans are naturally risk-averse and loss-averse, so we have become very creative in finding ways to distance ourselves from emotional pain. Two examples of how we can use a "flight" response to minimize and distance the feelings that arise from climate distress are "positive illusions" and "personal greenwashing."

Positive illusions and unrealistic optimism

The concept of positive illusions is part of a mental health model introduced in a 1988 paper by Shelley Taylor and Jonathon Brown. They suggest that there is a highly prevalent tendency for self-deception infused in our everyday thoughts that includes an inflated impression of our abilities and talents, persistent optimism about the future inconsistent with objective analysis, and an illusion of control. These tendencies help us cope with difficult and uncontrollable events and enhance self-esteem (Taylor and Brown 1988). However, it is easy to see how these inflated and distorted views can impair our decision-making.

Max Bazerman, a professor at Harvard Business School and Co-Director of the Center for Public Leadership at Harvard Kennedy School, feels strongly that the positive illusions of unrealistic optimism and the belief that events are more controllable than the facts dictate are two prominent dynamics that block our much-needed focus on climate change. We tend to believe that our own future will be brighter than other people's, and when we underestimate the risks in our lives, a psychological buffer is created that keeps us in an unrealistic comfort zone (Bazerman, Baron, and Shonk 2001).

Personal greenwashing

"Greenwashing" is a term generally used in marketing, when packaging or advertising text makes a product appear more environment-friendly than it actually is. One way we greenwash our lifestyle is when we become content with token efforts that make us feel better about ourselves but overinflate the actual degree of environmental benefit. While advertisers intentionally design with deception, our personal version tends to be much more innocent: it is an attempt to cope with and distance from the guilt and overwhelm of wanting to make change but not being ready or not knowing how. As the deeper feelings of grief and anxiety about climate change are worked through and emotional resiliency is cultivated, we are freed to take bolder steps toward change.

CLIMATE PSYCHOLOGY AND THE STRESS REACTION: FREEZE

Can you recall a time when someone said something unkind or shocking to you, and you were speechless until later, when you were then able to rehearse what you wish you had said? This mild deer-in-the-headlights reaction amplifies as the threat level increases. When people awaken to the realities of climate change, a persistent nowhere-to-run, nowhere-to-hide feeling of dread can make us feel intensely vulnerable, even terrorized. Freezing up—essentially dissociating—is the body and psyche's way to avoid this harrowing sense of overwhelm. It is also theorized that freezing has the adaptive benefit of allowing more time to devise an optimal response, although it is possible to be stuck in this state for prolonged periods (Mobbs *et al.* 2015). In the freeze response, the brain releases analgesics to sooth and numb out the psychic pain.

Ambivalence
While emotional reactions can freeze us in place, so can the cognitive dilemma of wanting to help the planet but also desiring the familiar creature comforts and ease of a lifestyle that may have a high carbon footprint. We like to keep our homes a comfortable temperature, fly to a favorite vacation spot, enjoy eating fresh fruit year-round; who wants to hear that we should sacrifice those entitlements? Renee Lertzman, Environmental Consultant and author of *Environmental Melancholia: Psychoanalytic Dimensions of Engagement*, describes it this way:

> What may inform these particular challenges to facing climate change through the lens of anxiety, conflict...may feel like double-binds. Arguably, we are becoming aware of the damaging impacts of our practices while being stitched into a way of life that can be hard to shift, creating extremely challenging psychological and social tensions tricky to navigate. (Lertzman 2015, p.1)

Prolonged cognitive and emotional freezing become procrastination as we find ourselves caught in a vortex of questions that never get answered: What is my role? Is there anything I can do? What are the changes I am willing to make? What are others doing? Will it make a difference? Is there enough time? While these questions are a normal part of emotional processing, they stall our forward momentum if they never get worked through.

In a similar way that we recognize the conflicting voices in our own heads, we can also hear these same voices gathered around the world's conference tables, creating ambivalence on the environmental policy level. The Fourth World Conservation Congress of the International Union for the Conservation of Nature, the world's largest environmental network, was tackling the issue of how to design conservation policies to address the impacts of climate change. While it was a rich gathering that identified a diverse array of clean-energy options, "Measurable change on this topic failed to materialize at this Congress..." and "Public expressions toward measurable changes in conservation policy...remain idle. We have argued that this observation is in part a consequence of a precautionary ambivalence, as well as value-based commitments to the existing framework" (Hagerman, Satterfield, and Dowlatabadi 2010, p.309). The same ambivalence that may be keeping us stuck is expressed and experienced both individually and collectively in the climate change arena.

Other psychological climate stress dynamics

In addition to the stress reactions that arise from our exposure to climate change, there are also other features at play that work against facing the challenge head-on. Anthony Leiserowitz, Director of the Yale Project on Climate Change Communication, states that, "You almost couldn't design a problem that's a worse fit with our underlying psychology or our institutions of decision-making" (Roewe 2015, p.1). While there are many theories about why disengagement from climate change action is so prevalent, here are five key perspectives.

1. HUMANS TEND TO PRIORITIZE IMMEDIATE CONCERNS OVER LONG-TERM CONSIDERATIONS

We have seen how our stress responses are wired to react to immediate threats—but climate change is not at all like confronting the proverbial saber-toothed tiger. In most parts of developed countries, the threat of climate chaos feels like it is off in a distant future. In all the ways that we are neurologically programmed to appraise threat, it does not really register. Our awareness tends to be fairly narrow, focused on keeping up with the concerns of our daily life and immediate pressures.

2. ABSTRACT DATA OFTEN DOES NOT TRANSLATE INTO PERSONAL CONCERN

Many things that contribute to climate change are not easy to see. For example, carbon dioxide, one of several greenhouse gas emissions, is invisible. We walk right through it all day, every day, blind to the many ways that it's entering the atmosphere. Anthony Leiserowitz adds, "You can look out the window right this very second, and there's CO_2 coming out of tailpipes, there's CO_2 coming out of buildings, there's CO_2 coming out of smokestacks, in fact there's CO_2 coming out of your mouth and nose this very second. But until I said it, you weren't conscious of it because it's invisible" (Roewe 2015, p.1). Because there is usually nothing in our immediate environment that is triggering a sense of urgency, we have to remind ourselves and actively remember what is happening— which increases the psychological challenge and weakens the prompts for daily eco-wise actions.

3. SOCIAL NORMING

We engage not just individually but also socially, routinely comparing our lifestyles and actions with those of others (Festinger 1954). Stanford University cites a study in which homeowners reduced their energy consumption if they were told they were using more than their neighbors (Mena-Werth 2016). Peer norms have a strong influence, and they can work in favor of change if our community is more eco-conscious or against change if an individual is "swimming against the current." If you are one of the first to have a heightened awareness of climate change, but you have personality traits that make you strongly averse to being pegged as an outsider or resist leadership roles, you may not be likely to initiate change.

4. DISSONANCE AND IDENTITY ISSUES

Per Espen Stoknes, author of *What We Think About When We Try Not to Think About Global Warming*, names dissonance and identity themes as key psychological barriers to understanding the impact of climate change.

He asserts that, "If there's a conflict between the facts, so to speak, and the values that guide my life, then my values will win" (Roewe 2015, p.1). This is part of a well-known cognitive and social psychology principle called "motivated reasoning." Essentially, people tend to seek out information that confirms their existing beliefs and ignore or minimize facts that oppose their positions. We cannot underestimate the strength of our ability to rationalize, and it occurs below our conscious awareness. When the beliefs that have helped us make sense of ourselves and the world are challenged, we can feel very threatened. In a conversation, this will often appear as stonewalling, argumentativeness, or simply shutting down and withdrawing.

5. EGALITARIAN VERSUS INDIVIDUAL WORLDVIEWS: WHOSE JOB IS IT TO FIX CLIMATE CHANGE?

While both top-down and bottom-up approaches are necessary in order to address the scale and complexity of climate change, some anti-government segments of the population with an inherent distrust of the government skirt environmental issues out of fear that the government might be required to take an active role (Kahan *et al.* 2012).

If it is up to the individual, it may feel like a foolish waste of time to recycle, take shorter showers, and walk rather than drive if it will not make a dent in the scale of what is occurring. Our thought process can go on to include a sense of things being unfair: "Why should I make sacrifices while corporate polluters continue to spew toxins into the air and water? I might as well enjoy life while I have the chance."

Healing directions

Clients who come into our practices and describe an increase in distress, with symptoms such as insomnia or ambient anxiety, may be having a visceral and unconscious response to the unsettling changes in the climate—even if they haven't experienced a direct, negative impact from a global-warming event. It's time to add a climate psychology lens to our intake and assessment approach. As therapists, we watch for constellations of symptoms that may indicate abuse or depression, and we can also begin to notice signs of climate-change-induced distress. It is part of our work to help clients "connect the dots" and gain insight into what is triggering their dis-ease, facilitate the appropriate emotional processing and cognitive restructuring, and develop new and healthy behavioral responses.

With our deepening understanding of the interconnectedness of all life, we can update our therapeutic goals to reflect an evolution of awareness that extends beyond personal fulfillment. We can now help our clients to heal in a direction that includes a good quality of life that is lived in harmony with the environment. This does not require an altruistic leap: it is ultimately pragmatic. We are witnessing on a global scale how individual and collective pursuits that are severed from the laws of nature have become dangerously unsustainable. There are growing examples of how global warming is compromising highly valued activities that are considered part of a desirable lifestyle: ski season is cut short because the snow levels reach record lows; public health officials are closing summer resorts with warnings of the hazards of toxic algae blooms in lakes and bays; a favorite seafood is no longer on the menu due to overfishing and marine "dead zones." These types of environmental impacts are escalating steeply in both number and kind. We could say that helping clients gain an understanding of the functional ecology of life *is* a way to achieve personal fulfillment: if they do not participate in protecting what they value, it will no longer be available to them.

Healing the self and healing nature become inseparable. As children we delight in splashing in mud puddles, finding animal-shaped clouds, and discovering the bugs and lizards that live under rocks. As adults, many vacations are planned so we can step outside of our busy lives and replenish ourselves in a natural environment. We relax when we hear the sound of the ocean and feel awe while watching a sunset or looking into the depths of the night sky. Most people inherently value and want to protect nature. Deep down inside, we recognize it as a part of us, as "home." As mental health professionals, when we help clients resolve their underlying distress, examine subconscious beliefs and assumptions, build resiliency, and connect more deeply within themselves and with others, it opens the gates for change and reparative engagement with the natural world.

As therapists, we also need to heal and participate in our connection with nature in order to help clients make the same connection. We live with the imperative to continue to build our integrity—clearly a lifelong endeavor, and who we are and how we live, along with our training, informs our therapeutic interventions. Not only will we be experiencing our own emotional reactions to climate issues, we also run the risk of secondary or vicarious trauma as we witness additional suffering and trauma in others. Kathy LeMay, CEO of Raising Change and author of *The Generosity Plan: Sharing your Time, Treasure and Talent to Shape the World*, expresses it this way:

> For people who work in social services and change and societal transformation, we decide we want to make a difference and enter this world fueled by hope and optimism... Then, day in and day out, years in and years out, [we experience] a few gains but what can feel like endless losses, [and] the uphill battle begins to take its toll... We hope we've made a difference... Partially because the losses are infuriating and partly because we weren't taught to grieve... We suppress the heartbreak... It could derail us and there is too much work to be done (LeMay 2016, p.1).

We need to face our losses as we discover the paths toward solutions. We can begin by greeting our clients—and ourselves—right where we are. Let us begin with an exploration of how resiliency can be cultivated as we awaken to our full human experience in the era of climate change.

Practices and perspectives: self-care for therapists

While the focus of this book is to offer methods and frameworks for helping clients with climate change issues, all of these approaches are valuable, perhaps essential, for us as therapists to experience as well. This is our human dilemma: we are all in this together.

There are seven perspectives that guide the work: connection, deep listening, creativity, presence, commitment, resolute compassion, and resiliency. They will be explored in depth in the upcoming chapters as we learn their very practical applications. Specific clarity and self-care practices designed for therapists, but also useful to clients, are listed on the worksheet at the end of this chapter. The seven perspectives described below may at first glance appear "soft" in their approach to a situation that calls for urgent and large-scale change. By looking more deeply, you will find that there is an essential fierceness—an unwavering stance that requires a clear mind, open heart, courage, and bold integrity. Cultivating these principles is like assembling the provisions essential for a long journey. These viewpoints can act as a guide for many valuable forms of expression, including education, leadership, advocacy, and community-building. Strong actions that embody these qualities have facilitated some of the greatest advances in human rights and life-affirming societal change. The first step is to begin with our own heart.

1. CONNECTION

Let an image form in your mind's eye of a web, the delicate filaments intricately connected, each one vibrating in response to the smallest movement on any part of the net. The web of life is a useful visual prompt for understanding interconnection as we explore climate change. This work requires that we feel the connecting strands between our deepest values, our gifts and talents, and our commitment to community and to nature. If we perceive differently, new ways of living will naturally emerge. As biochemist V. V. Rozinov elegantly states, "Look everywhere with your eyes, but with your soul never look at many things but at one" (Safransky 1990, p.148).

Experiencing interdependence guides our experience of being part of something larger than ourselves. As we recognize the living connections between ourselves and all other life forms, we begin to discover our role within the larger reparative movement. For example, you may be working with a client, an engineer with a speaking phobia, who is slated to address a 3,000-seat auditorium at a conference on climate solutions. If you help that person move through their fears and gain confidence in their public speaking, your role and theirs are linked, and both of you offer momentum to the forward direction of change. Perhaps someone in the audience now offers a contract to the engineer to install renewable energy devices, and another is inspired to mobilize an effort to green their workplace. The person who records and posts the video of the talk so it can reach an even larger audience plays a key role, as does the graphic designer who helped sell the tickets, as does the spouse who prepared lunch and offered encouragement to the keynote speaker. The sparks of inspiration expand through the connecting threads and into the hearts, minds, and actions of many. This movement needs artists, homemakers, scientists, economists, educators, indigenous wisdom holders, architects, students—all of us.

Tend and befriend

Fortunately, there is another stress response, one that is grounded in our connectedness. It is biologically just as old but not as widely known as the fight–flight–freeze trio. It is also an instinctual coping mechanism, but it can bring potential benefits to environment-triggered distress. Articulated by Dr. Shelley Taylor and her research team at the University of California, Los Angeles, it is known as "tend and befriend" (Taylor *et al.* 2000).

The "tend and befriend" principle arose from studies of the responses of mothers protecting their young during stressful situations; researchers observed that nurturing behaviors are actually triggered. It is theorized that the nurturing activities that "tend" to children stimulate oxytocin production, which is sometimes called the "love neurotransmitter" because it increases bonding and feelings of wellbeing (DeAngelis 2008). Oxytocin also leads people to increase and deepen their social contacts, the "befriend" part of the model.

While biologically it is a more natural female response—women are more likely than men to seek out social support—researchers reject the notion that our behaviors are solely driven by our biological gender. Rather, these findings point to a way that women can take the lead in modeling behaviors that can be just as "natural" and beneficial to men. When it comes to the long-term stressors that we see with climate issues, social networks are essential in order to bring forth new solutions, and it would be inaccurate to gender-type these helpful social groups (Azar 2000). As we will see, nurturance and connections are essential ingredients in this work.

2. Deep listening

This is both an internal and external practice. Here are two valuable ways to cultivate deep inner listening.

Listening within
Mindfulness
As therapists we are accustomed to helping clients understand their many inner voices: the self-talk of fear, the harsh inner critic, unexamined assumptions arising from childhood experiences disguised as truth. With mindfulness, a relatively new resource for psychotherapy, we can begin to find an expansive frame of mind with which to witness the parade of

thoughts, feelings, and sensations without engaging with them or pushing them away. It summons a nonjudgmental witnessing that can cultivate self-kindness, acceptance, and curiosity toward our own experiences.

When we pause mindfully, we have a moment to reflect and a greater ability to respond rather than react. We can identify more clearly the origins of our thinking habits. Our rumination is reduced and our ability to tolerate intense emotions increases, which is so valuable with environmental issues. The role of mindfulness within climate change psychology will be explored throughout the book.

Vision, dreams, and guided imagery

As we listen from a deeper place inside ourselves, below the chatter of the mind, we can also tap into wise insight, as natural and valid as the analytical part of our minds but underutilized in the industrialized West. Images are the language of this form of inner perception (Davenport 2009).

Changing our usual way of doing things requires re-visioning, an individual and collective seeing with fresh eyes our deep relationship with the web of creation. Ideas for creating new visions for transformation are emerging in many places simultaneously, from the jungles of the Amazon to policymakers in the United States.

In the early 1990s, Achuar shamans of Ecuador and Peru were sensing an imminent threat to their culture and land by oil companies they had not yet come into contact with. Through their dreams, they received guidance to seek out and create allies from the North. This partnership would enlist help to preserve their traditional ways of life, while also offer their healing gifts to an ailing world driven by overconsumption. From this vision the Pachamama Alliance, a non-profit organization headquartered in San Francisco, was born.

The Achuar shamans and elders describe the Western world as caught in a dreamlike trance, a nightmare, and the Pachamama Alliance now offers an "Awakening the Dreamer" educational program that has drawn participants from all 50 states in the United States and 81 countries and been translated into 16 languages, led by a team of close to 5,000 trained volunteer facilitators.[1] Noam Chomsky, well-known author and Professor Emeritus at Massachusetts Institute of Technology (MIT), agrees that indigenous cultures hold hope for our survival and are acting from much-needed visionary perspectives with climate change solutions. He states:

It's pretty ironic that the so-called 'least advanced' people are the ones taking the lead in trying to protect all of us, while the richest and most powerful among us are the ones who are trying to drive the society into destruction. (Keefer 2013, p.1)

When we listen to indigenous guidance, it does not mean that we are trying to imitate or transplant indigenous culture. Rather, many of these wisdom traditions have maintained vital stores of knowledge that we in the more developed world have lost through our focus on aggressive industrialization. As we reawaken to that wisdom, creative and evolving forms can flourish in our own communities.

The need for a new earth-honoring vision is also echoing in the halls of academia and public policy. Asim Zia, Director of the Institute for Environmental Diplomacy and Security at the University of Vermont, along with permaculturist Caitlin Waddick, describe it this way, "The Western vision of economic development through globalization, international trade, and conventional aid needs to be replaced with a place-based vision that emphasizes care for people, the Earth, and the future" (Zia and Waddick 2015).

Visions arise from silence, from deep listening. Inner listening has been a part of our human experience from our beginnings, and the practice and clarity within has been given a variety of names: "the still small voice," higher self, Satori, Dadirri, original nature, Osanubua, and many more. We are all visionaries, though most of us are out of practice. Methods for revitalizing this capacity are found throughout this book.

Listening to others

In order to reach the true heart of complex climate issues and engage in in-depth conversations, it is useful to develop a formidable center—an internal posture where we remain rooted in our own evolving, highest understanding, while also being truly receptive and flexible in hearing the experiences of others.

The notion of Beginner's Mind (*shoshin*) from Zen Buddhism is a useful guide. Our Beginner's Mind adopts an attitude of curiosity and openness, and a lack of preconceptions when we approach a topic, whether or not we are well educated in the subject (Suzuki 2006). The belief that we are "already an expert" is often accompanied by an intellectual arrogance that closes us off to valuable new perspectives.

As we respond to climate change concerns, our deep listening to others must also extend across disciplines. We need to bring this kind of genuine engagement to conversations with politicians, educators, engineers, indigenous elders, scientists—including all ages, races, and cultures. In the same way that biodiversity is essential for a healthy ecosystem, so are diverse perspectives necessary in order to generate life-affirming, inclusive, and comprehensive options.

3. CREATIVITY

Listening within is also the birthplace of imagination. Creativity shapes that which arises from our imagination into meaningful forms of expression. The threshold between our imagination and creative expression is familiar to anyone in the arts, but the door is open to everyone.

In the creative process, we bring our instincts and unedited intuition into relationship with the unknown, whether we are facing a blank canvas with a handful of paints, jotting notes for a speech on a napkin at the café, or in the scientific crowd, pondering how quantum gravity helps explain the origin of the universe. We send our inner critic on vacation and make room for messy, confusing bits and pieces of insight to swirl and shift before connecting in new and meaningful ways as we go with the creative process.

As we will discover, our creativity is supremely practical. As engineer, inventor, and cofounder of Sloan Kettering Hospital, Charles Kettering puts it, "Our imagination is the only limit to what we can hope to have in the future" (Sprenkle and Piercy 2005, p.195). Especially when we are called to navigate the myriad ways that climate change will require mitigation and adaptation, innovative approaches are essential. We are entering a new territory that demands new and creative solutions.

4. PRESENCE

In the estimated 500 billion galaxies (Howell 2014)—not stars or planets, but galaxies—there is only one you. No one else can offer the particular constellation of gifts and perspectives that your life journey has shaped. We are all welcome at the table. It begins with showing up, with being present. It does not require that we act in any particular way. We do not need to be other than ourselves; in fact, that would only work against us. But we do need to show up, because we are all needed in the circle. Dance legend Martha Graham expresses it elegantly:

> There is a vitality, a life force, an energy, a quickening that is translated through you into action, and because there is only one of you in all time, this expression is unique. And if you block it, it will never exist through any other medium and will be lost. (Kolb 2014. p.53)

As we become more present in ourselves and with others, an environment is created that calls forth the best qualities in each one of us and deepens our understanding of what is possible from ourselves and in the world.

5. COMMITMENT

Suggesting commitment can feel a bit edgy: commit to what, to whom? It is important to unhitch this principle from anyone else's idea of what you should be doing. Rather, commitment starts with an invitation to self-inquiry.

Cultural anthropologist Angeles Arrien tells a teaching story common among many traditional peoples. The story says that as we travel through life, we have two companions: Death and Destiny. We can use their whispers to launch our personal inquiry.

> Death continually asks us, "Are you using the great gift of life well? Destiny, on our right, is asking another question, "Are you doing what you've come here to do? Are you doing what you've come here to do?" (Arrien 2014)

How can we live a life that is in alignment with our clearest purpose? The answers will likely evolve throughout the different phases of our lives and find new channels of expression. They can come in any form and often emerge in our everyday moments and choices, creating a personal legacy of a life well lived. What do those choices look like, the ones that are true to you and also harmonious with an eco-friendly life?

Even with an abiding commitment, we are fallible and imperfect beings. It is challenging to remember and live out our intentions. This is our practice, and it requires many re-commitments and adjustments and much beginning again. We will bump up against our ambivalence and contradictions. Our goal is progress, not perfection, as we continue on our lifelong path. Perhaps we may be fortunate enough to experience wholeheartedness in our endeavors.

6. Resolute compassion

Engaging with climate disruption issues can touch some of our most vulnerable feelings. It may break our hearts over and over again, fill us with outrage, and cause us to sink into periods of despair as we learn more about what is happening to our world and how we got here. It may summon every raw feeling and raise mind-boggling questions.

Compassion contains an internal space large enough for every feeling. It makes room for us to be exactly where we are. It allows us to discover mental and emotional buoyancy and trust that we will not abandon the immensity and range of our feelings. The Dalai Lama puts it this way, "Love and compassion are necessities, not luxuries. Without them, humanity cannot survive" (Seaward 2011, p.94). The deeper meaning of how we engage in our lives cannot be measured by our titles or prestige, but rather by our growing integrity and depth of compassion.

7. Deep resiliency

What in us cannot be destroyed by the shadow side of human behavior or a superstorm, a fire, or drought? We might say that all the principles described here are resiliency practices: rediscovering and cultivating forms of inner strength that we may not realize already reside within us. We are cultivating the capacity to tolerate difficult feelings, which also expands our capacity to experience greater joy. Resiliency helps both therapists and clients to grow beyond their current comfort zone—to develop a fiercely compassionate and honest engagement with life. It is a challenging and fulfilling path.

Once again, Angeles Arrien draws on indigenous wisdom as she teaches us the questions a Shaman or elder would likely ask us when we are dispirited or disheartened. This is a helpful guide in our work:

When in your life did you stop singing?

When in your life did you stop dancing?

When in your life did you stop being enchanted by stories? Particularly, your own life story?

When did you stop finding comfort in the sweet territory of silence?

(Arrien 2014)

With climate disruption, there are so many things we do not know. Can we slow, halt, or reverse the damage that is impacting all species, cultures, and food and water supplies? As we dance with the unknown, we can still choose how to live our lives according to our truest values and in alignment with our place in the web of creation. I hear Rilke's statement as a useful prayer, and perhaps you will too, "May what I do flow from me like a river, no forcing and no holding back" (Macy and Brown 2014, p.209).

Additional resources

Davenport, L. (2009) *Healing and Transformation Through Self-Guided Imagery.* Berkeley, CA: Celestial Arts.

Hoggan, J. (2016) *I'm Right and You're an Idiot: The Toxic State of Public Discourse and How to Clean it Up.* Gabriola Island: New Society Publishers.

Marshall, G. (2015) *Don't Even Think About It: Why Our Brains are Wired to Ignore Climate Change.* New York, NY: Bloomsbury Publishing.

Vaughan-Lee, L. (ed.) (2013) *Spiritual Ecology: The Cry of the Earth.* Point Reyes Station, CA: The Golden Sufi Center.

WORKSHEET
Clarity and self-care

What would you like to do differently with respect to climate change issues?[2]

_____

_____

_____

_____

_____

What would happen if you *did not* make those changes?

_____

_____

_____

_____

What is the best thing you can imagine resulting from your participation in climate restoration efforts?

_____

_____

_____

_____

_____

Close your eyes for a moment and envision that positive outcome. Let it come to life in your imagination, noticing where you are and what you notice: the colors, textures, sounds, who is there, and especially how you feel. Where do you notice those feelings in your body? After a few moments, open your eyes.

What symbol or image can you use as a touchstone to reconnect you to this vision?

_____

What supports you in moving toward that vision?

_____

_____

_____

_____

What gets in the way?

_____

_____

_____

_____

Is there a step you are willing to commit to right now that would begin or enhance your participation?

_____

_____

_____

_____

_____

Close your eyes for a moment and begin to breathe into your heart. Imagine bringing that commitment into the center of your heart, and surround it and infuse it with your life force, a sense of "Yes!" and wellbeing. If it feels right, you can also place a hand over your heart for a few breaths. After a few moments, open your eyes.

Find a time this week to be in nature, whether it is a city park, your own backyard, or deep wilderness. When you are there, take a few moments to breathe in the fresh vitality of the natural environment, and breathe out gratitude for all the ways it sustains you. Let your eyes appreciate the colors and textures, your breath appreciate the freshness, your hands and feet the feel of solid support. Notice the ways that you are not in nature, but rather a part of it, sustained by the very same elements of air, water, the nutrients of the earth, and the fiery sun as the plants and trees.

Notes or drawing:

Chapter 2

Climate Change Grief

In 2015 the states of Oregon, Washington, New Jersey, Delaware, Texas, Oklahoma, Tennessee, Illinois, Mississippi, Arkansas, and Missouri suffered damage from severe flooding that included loss of life and property and shattered the peace of mind of those displaced from what they called home. At the same time, South Carolina had rain levels the likes of which they had not experienced in 1,000 years (McLeod 2015), and the South of France was struck by violent storms that left the area with apocalyptic scenes of devastation (Mullen 2015). Climate change is a global phenomenon, and our current trajectory points toward natural disasters—especially floods, fires, and storms—becoming ever more frequent and severe (Leaning and Guha-Sapir 2013).

In California, severe drought is impacting the primary farming communities in the Central Valley. In 2014, 500,000 acres of farmland lay fallow due to lack of water, with 17,000 seasonal and part-time jobs lost. Because of climate change, these numbers are predicted to increase each year, with no end in sight to the prolonged drought (Geiling 2015). With California producing most of the country's fruits, vegetables, and nuts, the shortage is being felt nationwide through increased food prices and reduced supply. In the Central Valley town of Okieville, neighbors rigged hoses from house to house to share the quickly diminishing underground water for their basic household needs (Crowder 2015).

From research on stress, we know that *any* change is considered a stressor, and today there are a multitude of fast-paced and often substantial shifts happening to more and more people, with even more severe changes on the horizon. As we saw in the previous chapter on climate change denial, many of us resort to ignoring the pain of loss by employing old, familiar psychological survival mechanisms. Just as our personal psychological defense patterns have a limited purpose, and generally work against us later in life, denial also fails to serve our collective distress. Fortunately, we can choose an alternate path, and we can begin by attending to our inner emotional landscape with awareness, honoring our natural physiological and psychological grief response as an organic way of moving through the pain, and transitioning to an empowered stance where we can make meaningful changes.

We come into this world equipped with a full palette of emotions[1] that color our life experiences, including but certainly not limited to sadness, joy, anger, wonder, fear, contentment, frustration, gratitude, confusion, and love. Yet we tend to reject the uncomfortable emotions, perhaps out of a belief that revealing them displays a weakness in our character, or a fear that intense feelings might consume us if not kept under wraps. We may view "negative" emotions as an obstacle to a good life. We have become very creative in finding methods to numb ourselves to the more thorny aspects of human experience: the full range of possible addictions includes relentless busyness, consumerism ("retail therapy"), media absorption, mindless over eating and drinking, and recreational/ prescription drugs. We are not taught how to cultivate our emotional intelligence, benefit from the meanings our emotions carry, or recognize how they naturally flow and change.

Our crafty strategies for avoiding pain come at a high price. It is not the emotions themselves but our turning away from them that damages us—as well as others and the environment around us. When our normal emotional responses are suppressed, they transform into toxic pockets of pain that seep into and poison our health, our relationships, and many other aspects of our lives. Unresolved distress that gets buried can also be like a landmine: when triggered, it erupts in distorted ways. Discarded grief can sink into depression. Suppressed fear can disguise itself as anger.

Living in an endangered world is shifting our collective human consciousness. Nearby rivers that were once enjoyed for their beauty become dangerous when they threaten to flood our community or become polluted. When summers get hotter and longer, there can grow an eerie unease toward what formerly provided us with comfort in the welcome rhythms of the seasons. *How can we open our eyes, hearts, and minds to the losses associated with climate change without sinking into despair?*

By living through the grief and trusting that we will not break, even when our hearts do. By living our lives according to our deepest values.

By becoming part of the solution.

Grief flows, and when we emerge on the other side of the process we are often clearer, stronger, and more resilient than before.

Five stages of climate grief

"Disenfranchised grief" is a term used to describe losses and sorrow that there are no socially prescribed methods for engaging or acknowledging. While it usually refers to the anguish that can accompany conditions like infertility, or the heartache many feel over the death of a beloved pet (Doka 2002), it is highly relevant to climate change grief. The widespread denial of climate change losses prevents our emotional pain from being socially acknowledged and validated. Those touched by this grief may be viewed as overly sensitive, as exaggerating the issue, or even as emotionally unbalanced. These responses can encourage individuals to isolate, remain silent, and become disenfranchised from their own grief process, rather than move through it with support.

Steve Running, Regents Professor at the University of Montana and one of the authors of the Intergovernmental Panel's Report on Climate Change, is helping to articulate the natural climate-induced mourning process, and he developed the model "Five Stages of Climate Grief," building on the work of Elizabeth Kübler-Ross (Running 2007).

STAGE ONE: DENIAL

The first stage, denial, can persist for a long time, as we have seen in the previous chapter. Even with the staggering intensity of the environmental disasters around us, climate change ranked near the bottom of policy concerns among United States citizens (Riffkin 2014). But even denial can serve a time-limited psychological purpose. Poet David Whyte describes a beautiful and compassionate perspective on how denial—or in his words "hiding"—can be useful and beautiful.

Hiding is a way of holding ourselves until we are ready to come into the light. Hiding is one of the brilliant and virtuoso practices of almost every part of the natural world: the protective quiet of an icy northern landscape, the held bud of a future summer rose, the snow bound internal pulse of the hibernating bear. Hiding is underestimated... Hiding is creative, necessary and beautifully subversive of outside interference and control. Hiding leaves life to itself, to become more of itself. Hiding is the radical independence necessary for our emergence into the light of a proper human future. (Whyte 2015, pp.113–115)

While all the stages of grief are natural, it is essential to the healing process to feel the flow of the grief process and avoid becoming stuck in any one phase.

STAGE TWO: ANGER

In stage two of Running's climate grief model, people get angry. They can become indignant at the notion of changing their desirable and often hard-earned lifestyle. This stage is characterized by inflammatory statements like, "I refuse to live in a treehouse in the dark eating nuts and berries" (Running 2007, p.1). Inflating what could be reasonable lifestyle changes to the level of the absurd is another way of pushing away reality and guarding against experiencing our feelings.

Anger and sadness are closely paired, with one often layered beneath the other. It is easier for some personalities to default to sadness, while others habitually lean into anger. Those who have difficulty tolerating emotional vulnerability are more likely to lash out. If an individual is feeling weak or powerless, anger can make them feel stronger. Others feel threatened by the possibility of standing up for themselves, and so have developed a greater tolerance for emotional pain: they are more comfortable living in sadness.

STAGE THREE: BARGAINING

As people move into stage three, bargaining, they may no longer deny changes in the climate but they grasp for positive news and vigorously ignore the negative reports. There is a pervasive attitude of "It's not so bad." This belies a faulty belief that we are exempt from the most significant impacts, that we will just "ride it out." We may even introduce a positive spin: "England will be a new wine-growing region, as their area is predicted to become more Mediterranean. It will be fun to try those new wines" (Vidal 2013, p.1). In this stage we are also prone to making token environmental efforts, the "greenwashing" described in Chapter 1.

Those who take this stance are often coming from a place of unexamined class and racial privilege. Climate change magnifies and intensifies existing inequality and has a greater impact on people of color, low-income families, and indigenous communities. These impacts include unjust financial burdens, increased health risks, and social and cultural disruptions (Lynn, MacKendrick, and Donoghue 2011). Those populations cannot afford new technologies to mitigate the effects or easily move to a more desirable area. Naomi Klein, award-winning journalist and author of *This Changes Everything: Capitalism vs. the Climate*, clearly illuminates the issue:

> If wealthy white Americans had been left without food and water for days in a giant stadium after Hurricane Katrina, would it be possible for so many Republican politicians to deny the crisis? If Australia were at risk of disappearing and not large parts of Bangladesh, would Prime Minister Tony Abbott feel free to extol the burning of coal as "good for humanity?" If Toronto were being battered by historic typhoons that cause mass evacuations and not Tacloban in the Philippines, would building tar sands pipelines still be the centerpiece of Canada's foreign policy? (Klein 2014, p.1)

Chris Boeskool (2016) translates privilege into simple terms:

> Equality can *feel* like oppression. But it's not. What you're feeling is just the discomfort of losing a little bit of your privilege—the same discomfort that an only child feels when she goes to preschool and discovers that there are other kids who want to play with the same toys as she does. (p.1)

Fearing the loss of privilege can be another powerful driver of climate denial. As mental health professionals, we can assist clients from a privileged background with examining the underlying biases that contribute to climate-related inequality. We can listen, validate, and learn from disadvantaged clients and help them discover what empowerment will mean for them. Whatever background we come from as mental health professionals will give us useful tools for assisting all types of clients as we examine our own biases. These considerations play a significant role in correcting social imbalance and generating fair and reasonable solutions.

STAGE FOUR: DEPRESSION

According to Running, depression sets in when we face climate change squarely but then feel overwhelmed by the scope of the problem. The scale and complexity of climate issues can make us feel hopeless, as though any meaningful change is impossible. There are many scientists and activists who succumb to melancholy when clean-energy policies are delayed and there is a shift from aiming for prevention to planning for adaptation (Richardson 2015). A professor of ocean geology wept during a radio interview while discussing the rapid changes that are being measured in the seas. She fears that by the end of the century her own daughters will not have the opportunity to see coral reefs or enjoy shellfish—the rich ocean life that we've always taken for granted (Harrabin 2015). Some climate scientists have even begun describing "pre-traumatic" stress disorder; they experience overwhelm and intrusive thoughts when they look to a future that promises increasing environmental catastrophes (Holmes 2015).

STAGE FIVE: ACCEPTANCE

Running describes acceptance as a stage where people calmly acknowledge the realities of climate change and begin exploring options for participating in clean-energy solutions. In the most recent literature, new models of the stages of grief have shifted from describing a linear progression through the stages to a process that functions more like a wheel. We often slide back and forth among the feelings that predominate in the various stages. It is normal to reach some degree of acceptance but then slide back into depression or bargaining for a while. Educating clients about the stages of grief and the likely fluctuation in their emotional progress gives them an internal roadmap and normalizes their feelings. It can be much easier to bear the intense feelings if we know that there is the possibility of resolution.

The sanctity of pain

Many wisdom traditions hold the perspective that "open alertness that allows our heart to be stirred by the suffering of others is appreciated as a strength" (Macy and Johnstone 2012, p.67). Opening our hearts to the pain of others touches us at the very root of what it is to be human. Empathy, the vicarious experiencing of the thoughts, feelings, and attitudes of others, is a beautiful initial step toward deeply engaging the grief caused by climate change.

However, there is a downside to empathy. Olga Klimecki, a psychologist and neuroscientist at the University of Geneva, points out that, "When we share the suffering of others too much, our negative emotions increase. It carries the danger of an emotional burnout" (Hoffman 2013, p.1). Instead we can cultivate compassion, which actually builds emotional resiliency as we attend to the suffering in ourselves and others.

EMPATHY VERSUS COMPASSION

While the terms are defined differently among psychologists, the meaning of empathy used here is found reflected in the familiar proverb, "Walk a mile in my shoes." We enter the pain of another, experiencing it as though it were our own. Our empathetic responses stimulate brain activity in the anterior insula and anterior medial cingulate cortex, a neural network connected to pain and unpleasantness (Fan *et al.* 2011). Our own nervous system attunes to the experience of another, and we absorb their pain. It is as if a person is drowning and reaches out for help, and we jump in to assist them and go under too.

In contrast, researchers define compassion as "feeling concern for another's suffering and desiring to enhance that individual's welfare" (Goetz, Keltner, and Simon-Thomas 2010, p.351). There remains a sense of space, a boundary, between our experience and the other person, but it does not interfere with deep connection and authentic care. Compassion training increases activity in the medial orbitofrontal cortex, putamen, pallidum, and ventral tegmental area, brain regions involved in emotional regulation and positive emotions (Klimecki *et al.* 2013). A compassionate response releases the peptide hormone oxytocin, which is associated with love and connection. The oxytocin then triggers the neurotransmitter dopamine, a feel-good "reward," and the calming neurotransmitter serotonin (Keltner, March, and Smith 2010). Cultivating compassion increases our altruistic behavior, and we can have an openhearted, genuine, caring response without absorbing the pain.

It could appear that maintaining boundaries and differentiation could create an "us versus them" mentality, but with an open mind and heart we know that at any time the great wheel of life can turn. Our roles are not fixed: the caregiver can quickly become the one in need, and the person previously struggling can shift into a supportive role. The most authentic work is grounded in our knowing that we are all part of the same life; one that brings a constant flow of fluctuating circumstances. We can begin with an empathetic understanding, and stand on a compassionate foundation.

Research shows that compassion can be taught, and with regular practice it begins to train our neural network to make compassion our new baseline response. The most-studied compassion training is the Buddhist *Metta* practice, a practice of lovingkindness. The steps for learning *Metta* can be found on the worksheet in Chapter 6.

Moving through climate change grief with emotional resiliency

Grief is a form of love: we grieve the loss of what made us feel most deeply connected. With climate change grief, it may be loss of the dream of a future for your grandchildren free of the challenges that are currently emerging. Perhaps it is a loss of innocence with respect to our country's local or national political structure. It can include the devastating loss of lives and property. Whatever the scope, level, or intensity of the loss, the process of grieving evokes the same emotional phases. While everyone grieves in their own way and time, here are five tools that build resiliency and cultivate a compassionate field for experiencing all facets of the grief process. They are trust, kind curiosity, somatic awareness, knowing the story, and creative expression.

TRUST

The very act of trusting the grief process and our natural flow of emotions has great power. While there may be moments that are difficult to bear and at times may seem never-ending, our feelings do in fact shift and move. It can be helpful to recall a time in the past when you navigated a loss and came through the other side. This will enhance your trust in your own capacity to abide with the experience of significant loss. This kind of trust deepens our capacity to embrace all of life and tolerate the full range of intense emotions.

KIND CURIOSITY

Try an experiment: meet all your feelings as though they are unfamiliar guests in your home. Greet them and try to find out all about them. What are they saying? What do they want? This approach creates a welcome sense of inner spaciousness, because one part of you acts as host and other parts experience the feelings. When you can witness your emotions in this way, without condemnation or approval, it helps build your core emotional strength, and you become less prone to being overwhelmed by feelings. Sinking into the feelings or pushing them away often amplifies their intensity, and we dig neurological grooves that trap us in emotional loops. Cultivating the ability to observe our emotional "visitors" without self-judgment or reaction helps us release old habits and opens us to a world of self-discovery.

SOMATIC AWARENESS

The pain of grief inhabits the body as well as the mind and emotions. We develop somatic awareness by paying attention to the ways that feelings manifest in the body: Is there a heaviness in the chest? A knot in the stomach? A clenching of the jaw? Recognizing the somatic expressions of our feelings helps us know where to direct self-soothing. Think of how you might calm a pet or young child who has been startled by a loud noise. You can turn that kind attentiveness to your own distress. Step away from the busyness of your day for a few moments and place a loving hand over your own heart or belly. You could remind your jaw how to relax with the natural releasing quality and awareness of the out-breath, and simply pausing can bring you more directly into the present moment.

KNOWING THE STORY

What are the beliefs that narrate your grief? "It's my fault. It's someone else's fault. This will never end. I can't bear it. I deserve this. I don't deserve this. We're out of time. We're doomed. I'm too small to make a difference." The unexamined stories we repeat to ourselves are almost always distorted. There may be elements of truth, but we amplify, minimize, add layers of self-judgment, and efficiently filter out relevant and often positive aspects of the situation.

We can begin by questioning our own thoughts. "Is what I'm saying to myself really accurate? Can I be certain? What else is true? Are any of these statements relevant? I can learn and gain strength from overcoming challenges. I have something to contribute to making the world a better place. Positive change is possible. I'm willing to try."

Changing our inner narrative is not intended to impose superficial peace. By loosening our investment in our story, fresh perspectives and other feelings can naturally arise in the space that is created. This kind of self-inquiry cultivates a more balanced and realistic view. There is a wonderful Cherokee story[2] that illustrates how parts of ourselves can compete with one another and the importance of our conscious relationship to our inner voices and drives.

> An old Cherokee is teaching his grandson about life. "A fight is going on inside me," he said to the boy. "It is a terrible fight and it is between two wolves. One is…anger, envy, sorrow, regret, greed, arrogance, self-pity, guilt, resentment, inferiority, lies, false pride, superiority and ego." He continued, "The other is…joy, peace, love, hope, serenity, humanity, kindness, benevolence, generosity, truth, compassion, and faith. The same fight is going on inside you—and inside every other person, too." The grandson thought about it for a minute and then asked his grandfather, "Which wolf will win?" The old Cherokee simply replied, "The one you feed" (Scott 2012, p.1).

We can begin inquiring into what beliefs and assumptions we are feeding ourselves and dwelling on—about our experience, our capacity, the reality of climate change, and the very nature of our interconnected life.

CREATIVE EXPRESSION

We become immobilized when we sink into despair. That may be why almost all grief rituals around the world include music and storytelling. Expressing feelings outwardly through writings, drawing, movement, and action is a powerful way of assimilating thoughts, feelings, and sensations of grief and can propel us into a time of rebuilding. When we move through the grief process, we can convert our distress into passion for effective action. As we begin to express our thoughts, feelings, and behavior in alignment with our deepest values, we build tremendous strength and resiliency. We find ways to attend to our own integrity in spite of what others may do or say. With climate change, we can shift from the disempowered position of "What have we done?!" to a passionate "What can we do?"

Evolutionary transformation

Our challenge, responsibility, and participation can go far beyond a calmer acceptance and simple actions. We can recognize that we are living in an era in the evolution of humanity and all the species on this earth that has never been experienced before. We can awaken to our unprecedented role individually and systemically, participating in intentional evolution toward a sustainable culture for all of life. Cosmologist Brian Swimme summarizes it this way:

> We are living on the planet at the time when the evolutionary dynamics are changing. And the simple way of saying it is that they're changing from genetic determination to cultural determination... That is an amazing new power that's taking place on the planet. We, then, have to confront the fact that this planet is evolving according to our decisions... Our responsibility is to structure the human presence on the planet so the fundamental conditions of life are strong and vibrant, and carry into the future. (Swimme 2007)

Swimme is speaking to the science of what is occurring on our planet, and many other disciplines—engineering, education, philosophy, and, in our case, psychology—can align to this new reality and become part of the transformation. This is a remarkable era in the evolution of life on earth. It requires a reshaping of our ethics toward an interspecies awareness and a global perspective. Our enjoyment of our individual freedoms can no longer be severed from their impact on the web of life. Once we move through the grief process, we can inhabit our place of belonging within the whole of life.

Additional resources

Greenspan, M. (2004) *Healing Through the Dark Emotions: The Wisdom of Grief, Fear and Despair*. Boston, MA: Shambhala Publications.

Klein, N. (2014) *This Changes Everything: Capitalism vs. the Climate*. New York, NY: Simon and Schuster.

Lertzman, R. (2015) *Environmental Melancholia: Psychoanalytic Dimensions of Engagement*. New York, NY: Routledge.

Stang, H. (2014) *Mindfulness and Grief*. New York, NY: CICO Books.

WORKSHEET
Mapping your grief journey and exploring privilege

Self-inquiry: climate grief

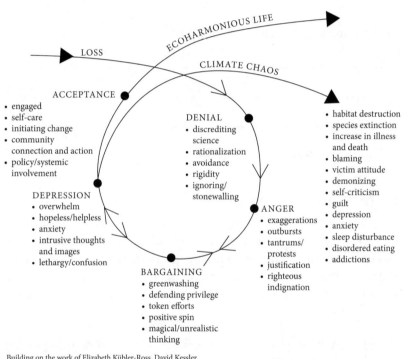

ECOHARMONIOUS LIFE

LOSS

CLIMATE CHAOS

ACCEPTANCE
- engaged
- self-care
- initiating change
- community connection and action
- policy/systemic involvement

DENIAL
- discrediting science
- rationalization
- avoidance
- rigidity
- ignoring/ stonewalling

DEPRESSION
- overwhelm
- hopeless/helpless
- anxiety
- intrusive thoughts and images
- lethargy/confusion

ANGER
- exaggerations
- outbursts
- tantrums/ protests
- justification
- righteous indignation

BARGAINING
- greenwashing
- defending privilege
- token efforts
- positive spin
- magical/unrealistic thinking

- habitat destruction
- species extinction
- increase in illness and death
- blaming
- victim attitude
- demonizing
- self-criticism
- guilt
- depression
- anxiety
- sleep disturbance
- disordered eating
- addictions

Building on the work of Elizabeth Kübler-Ross, David Kessler, Yukon Hospice, and Steve Running.

CLIMATE CHANGE GRIEF WHEEL

Take time to reflect about where you are on the climate change grief wheel. Write about it, and note the things you are experiencing that help you recognize which phase you are currently in.

What do you need right now in order to experience this phase fully, and what will support the flow of the grief process?

_____

_____

_____

_____

How can you acquire that kind of support?

_____

_____

_____

_____

Beginning to examine privilege

This is an opportunity to begin reflecting about the ways that our social, economic, racial, gender, and cultural filters influence our views and opportunities. When it comes to climate change, inner and outer dialogues that help us evolve toward more compassion and equity are profoundly impactful on personal, community, and international policy levels.

Do you see yourself as part of a privileged or a disadvantaged group?

_____

What sorts of things do you take for granted when it comes to resources related to climate change?

_____

_____

_____

Ask—how are my experiences different from other groups? Why do the differences matter? How do they play out in the real world?

_____

_____

_____

_____

_____

_____

_____

_____

Close your eyes and take a moment to imagine what it might be like as a member of a different group than your own.

   Imagine what your life would be like if you shared your privilege.
   What possibilities can you see without your privilege?[3]

Notice your reactions, and write about them.

_____

_____

_____

_____

_____

_____

_____

_____

Chapter 3

An Overview of Clinical Themes Involving Climate Change

Amy's story[1]

I've been on edge for a few days now, hearing the news that a hurricane, building in strength just off the coast, may be headed our way. I've already lived through many false warnings of big storms. I even enjoy heavy downpours when my pair of thick socks are clean and there's still a packet of instant hot chocolate in the cabinet. But I can't help but try to mentally record the strength of the wind on the way to the store, and I haven't gone to sleep the last couple nights without picturing the anchorman's drawings of possible storm trajectories. Should I pack up, just in case? Head to my sister's for the weekend? My neighbor, Jack, who has grown up in this town, said he knows these winds inside out. They speak to him, and he shakes his head, "Amy, these are *not* the kind of storms to worry about."

As I get home for the night, I wrap the reassurance of old Jack's voice around me and settle in to be lulled by the flickering blue light of the TV—any old rerun will do. Maybe the sound of the wind and rain was making Dixon slow to wind his way onto my lap and purr, but we finally both landed.

I jump each time a sharp gust rattles the windows, momentarily sending Dixon flying. Is the water sluicing down the window pane a warning? I tire myself out from repetitious worry and bully myself with a "Just go to bed" command. I obey. I pop three NyQuil and silently pray for rest.

Suddenly it's happening.

The banging is loud. Time is scrambled. My head aches. It's dark except for rhythmic flashes of blue and red lights. A horn blares garbled announcements. Extra-large men with flashlights, ropes, and wet yellow jackets surround me. The rain is sideways in my house. I grab a photo and my hairbrush off the table. Where's Dixon? I'm being pushed, I think. "Move. NOW!"

I can't tell if I fell, but I'm in a van. The metal bench is hard, the air thick. It's hard to draw a breath as the bumpy road rattles our bones. My knee is aching and I look at my leg as though I'm peering down from on top of a roof. I see a small, crimson kneecap with pretty, lacy red threads. Where's my Dixon? Someone I don't recognize is sitting beside me in the van. They open their mouth, but nothing comes out.

* * *

It's been almost two days, I think, and I get to return home briefly. I've been warned that there's been lots of damage—I can't move back in yet, but I can gather some of my things. Nothing prepares me for what I see.

I'm being driven into a boggy hell that I don't recognize. I really can't take it in as the place where I've loved my favorite routines for years— Meg's Cookhouse for coffee, part-time work at Front Street Books, my cozy little cottage—now rubble. My mind keeps falling through trap doors underneath my thoughts as I try to understand what I'm seeing. My legs are heavy as I walk past a mattress soaked in a briny, sour mash of gasoline and dark water. There is part of a car wedged between tree branches like an avant-garde art installation. Other trees are downed, and there are intermittent piles of lumber that I realize are pieces of homes.

Without the familiar landmarks, it takes a while for me to find the place that used to be mine. The sunlight catches a small mosaic of grey glass on the floor, all that remains of my TV. I stare, puzzled by how the glass remained, since large pieces of furniture, roof, and walls were torn and carried away by the winds. My mind finds pleasure latching on to the little puzzles, since it can't grasp the enormity of what has happened. I see a favorite green sock, half of my birthday gift from my grandmother, wedged part way under a piece of wood. While I recognize it, it is no longer familiar. I can hear someone sobbing nearby but I don't want to see who it is.

Multiple losses and complex grief

If we now imagine Amy coming into our therapy practice, we can easily assess layers of multiple losses and consider the clinical themes that may emerge. On a physical level, she has lost her home, job, financial security, and, at least temporarily, her social structure. It is unclear in this storm scenario whether there was also loss of lives in this community. In addition, we do not know if she will be reunited with her cat, Dixon, or if he suffered injuries. The severe and multiple losses could lead to a complex and prolonged bereavement process.

Amy may blame herself for not heeding the warning signs. While it appears she was operating from a "normalcy bias" that is common in disaster situations, she may now lose trust in her judgment or instincts and feel shame for putting herself and her pet in harm's way. Many communities are caught off guard by the intensifying relationship to nature that climate change is creating. With Hurricane Katrina, there was a failure of over 50 levees and flood walls, allowing tens of billions of gallons of water to surge into vast areas of New Orleans, killing close to 2,000 people and damaging 90,000 square miles. While there are many reasons the levees broke, this was an unanticipated outcome in an area very familiar with hurricanes (Mittal 2005).

Amy's account of the event has confusing gaps in the details and timing of what occurred. It is unknown whether she suffered a concussion from a fall or flying debris and/or disassociation. She may want to try and reconstruct what happened. What were her preexisting conditions? With the use of NyQuil for insomnia, are there addiction issues?

Amy may develop symptoms of post-traumatic stress disorder that are triggered by the sound of rain or rattling windows. Perhaps she no longer trusts people, like her neighbor Jack, someone who had previously been a faithful source of comfort and advice.

Her spiritual, religious, or existential beliefs may be plagued with doubts: Why did this happen? What does it say about God, life, nature?

If governments or people are partly to blame for the intensity of climate disasters, she may be challenging her ideas about human nature in ways that had never been called into question before.

While there have always been natural disasters—earthquakes, floods, hurricanes, droughts, blizzards, tornados—changes in the climate are producing much more frequent extreme weather events. While scientists cannot always correlate particular storms to climate change, they do recognize the increase in the number and intensity of natural disasters as an outcome of global warming.[2] Natural disasters of all kinds have increased by 430 percent since 1975 (Klein 2007). The frequency of Category 4 and 5 hurricanes has almost doubled around the world since 1970, and scientists are now considering whether to add a Category 6, since the velocities of recent storms have far surpassed the top of the Saffir-Simpson scale, which categorizes storms based on wind speed. It is difficult to comprehend the implications of needing to extend this scale, given that Hurricane Katrina came ashore as a Category 3 (Blakemore 2006).

Communal response

While Amy's experience contains features common among those directly touched by environmental disasters, everyone experiences traumatic loss and recovery in their own way and in their own time. There are many factors that influence this, and a few key components are core resiliency, attachment style, amount and type of support following the incident, the number of losses connected to the event, duration of high distress, degree of violence, and whether the loss was unexpected.

Both the impact and healing from climate change disasters are not just individual experiences: there is also collective trauma. Consider how many other stories of loss could be told in Amy's town. Whenever possible, reuniting community is essential to healing grief. We explored in the introduction how interconnected our beliefs and actions are with the environment, and these connections remain essential in the healing process as well. Inside/outside, self/community/environment can no longer be treated in silos.

When a community can recall their experiences together, in a safe space, the past becomes a collective story of grief, and compassionate bonds help build emotional buoyancy among members, helping to facilitate the healing process. It would serve Amy tremendously not only to receive individual psychotherapy, but also to experience solidarity with her neighbors and become empowered by actively being a part of community restoration. The next chapter explores the stages of disaster recovery and guidelines for rebuilding community.

Without minimizing the profound suffering and trauma that accompanies devastating loss, it is not uncommon for individuals and communities to also experience powerful redemptive moments in the aftermath of a disaster. This is an intricate and tender subject. It is essential to avoid using veiled platitudes when there is a right and a need to grieve. There can be no expectation of epiphanies. Yet at times, along with grief, there is a deep satisfaction in responding well to an emerging situation—both through the creative strength and agency of providing what is needed and experiencing generosity and altruism from others. There can be a spontaneous rising up of impromptu kitchens and shelters within affected areas. Neighbors often serve as unofficial first responders (Solnit 2009).

Communities demonstrate remarkable tenacity and resiliency in addressing the destructive effects of a disaster. There is freedom within the social interactions that "fulfills many of the essential human needs that are missing in the everyday life of modern society" (Fritz 1996, pp.27–78). There can be a self-defined restructuring of roles, where previous status or racial barriers give way to a more humanitarian focus (Klausner and Kincaid 1956), and there is a temporary democratization of the civil structure. These shifts can stimulate hope of correcting old injustices. Rebecca Solnit, author of *A Paradise Built in Hell*, expresses it this way:

> The history of disaster demonstrates that most of us are social animals, hungry for connection, as well as for purpose and meaning… [Disasters] are a crack in the walls that ordinarily hem us in, and what floods in can be tremendously destructive—or creative. (Solnit 2009, p.305)

I would add that both are generally in the mix, with creativity prompted by necessity. Solnit goes on to say that this kind of induced change can introduce us to a different kind of society, one that may include gift economies, sharing resources, a kinder and more intimate way of relating. Priorities get recalibrated and a deeper purpose comes into focus with a united communal effort. She goes on:

The joy in disaster comes, when it comes, from the purposefulness, the immersion in service and survival, and from an affection that is not private and personal but civic: the love of strangers for each other, of a citizen for his or her city, of belonging to a greater whole, of doing the work that matters. (p.306)

Sociologist Charles Fritz also affirms that large-scale disasters can produce mentally healthy conditions. He posits that:

In everyday life many human problems stem from people's preoccupation with the past and the future, rather than the present... Disasters provide a temporary liberation from the worries, inhibitions, and anxieties associated with the past and the future because they force people to concentrate their full attention on immediate moment-to-moment, day-to-day needs... [A disaster] speeds the process of decision-making [and] facilitates the acceptance of change... (Fritz 1996, pp.61–62)

If we eliminate his references to disasters and read only the parts about releasing past and future thoughts and finding freedom in bringing full attention to the present moment, we might think he was describing mindfulness practice. Disasters, surprisingly, can initially foster many of the conditions of mindful awareness: a reduction in preconceived notions, heightened vibrancy toward life, a shift to a present-moment focus. As we will see in the next chapter on treatment approaches, mindfulness can also be brought to climate crises in our proactive movements toward renewable and regenerative living, when treating acute trauma from climate-change-related disasters, and in long-term healing and recovery.

While these resiliency trends are validated in numerous disaster research studies, we are on new ground with climate-change-related events. In the past, a tornado or flood were usually singular or rare incidents, and there people found satisfaction in coming together to rebuild their community. With climate change, there is a persistent threat because the frequency, intensity, and geographic range of climate-change-induced destruction is on the rise. The annual rise in global temperatures cannot be resolved with familiar tactics. We will need deeper psychological resiliency and more radical adaptation to meet the severity of the challenges ahead.

Psychotherapy to facilitate transformation

Treatment and healing in the context of climate change mean more than simply helping people cope with loss. They can include co-creating new individual and collective stories of evolutionary transformation, as Swimme describes in Chapter 2. Some environmental leaders go so far as to call our current climate transition a requiem (Hamilton 2010), an elegy for the dying of many of the ways we have known life, including the extinction of species, as we exit the Holocene and enter into the Anthopocene era (Kolbert 2014). But this transition is not just about loss: we can also become midwives who aid in the birth of new possibilities.

This liminal period is filled with potential, and it has been given many names, including the "Great Turning" (Macy and Johnstone 2012) by general systems theorist and Buddhist scholar Joanna Macy, along with David Korten, former professor of the Harvard Business School. Thomas Berry, Catholic priest and cultural historian, calls it the "Great Work": "The Great Work now…is to carry out the transition from a period of human devastation of the Earth to a period when humans would be present to the planet in a mutually beneficial manner" (Berry 1999, p.3).

Recovery from climate change disasters can no longer be about returning to "normal," even though there is an intense pull to seek out familiar comforts. It may literally be impossible to rebuild some homes and communities in the same areas if, for example, there is ongoing flooding due to a permanent rise in the sea level. As old structures are uprooted, we are offered the opportunity to sow new ways of being that will shift humanity's thinking, acting, and forward momentum.

We all become attached to the full spectrum of our routines—the healthy as well as the dysfunctional. Disruption from climate change disasters can breach our habitual attachment to the familiar and move us toward a conscious commitment to deeper values and an evolving sense of purpose. We are presented with fresh choices, and we can choose to live with a grounded awareness in a sustainable lifestyle that is aligned with our growing consciousness of the impact of our actions on the environment and other beings.

Regenerative development, systemic sustainability

As mental health professionals, we know that change is difficult and complex. Change of any kind is a stressor, many of which are measured on the Holmes and Rahe Stress Inventory. Climate change causes stress in every structure: economic, health, political policy, technology, city planning, agriculture, architecture, education, personal lifestyle, and philosophy. It may seem naïve to view such radical changes in positive terms. Yet history shows us through countless examples—from the medical revolution through the renaissance to women's right to vote—that collective beliefs and actions can and do change. In Chapter 6, we will read about communities in different parts of the world that have increased their lifestyle satisfaction, either following a climate change disaster or by proactively creating a new model of transformative community. While it is not an easy path, the greatest catalyst for transformation is often crisis.

Milton Friedman, an American economist who received the 1976 Nobel Memorial Prize in Economic Sciences, observed that "only a crisis—actual or perceived—produces real change. When that crisis occurs, the actions that are taken depend on the ideas that are lying around. That, I believe, is our basic function: to develop alternatives to existing policies, to keep them alive and available until the politically impossible becomes politically inevitable" (Friedman 2002, p.xiv).

Because climate change catastrophes impact entire communities, regions, and even countries, such as the Maldives, which is predicted to be completely under water in 30 years (Christ 2016), they are ultimately global issues, needing the skills and talents of our global human community. We all rely on the same biosphere. There is not a single or simple vision of how the new systems will look or function. Some leaders point toward a back-to-nature model, with locally sourced foods and cooperative economies. Others describe a highly technological future, where we utilize renewable sources of energy to speed up modes of transportation and information in fast-paced urban settings. The ways individuals and communities rebuild will probably look different based on factors like the existing culture, political drivers, and natural resources in each area. Given our planet's diverse geographic and cultural regions, fundamental principles are being discovered that will support a broad range of transformative options. One such set of principles is "regenerative development," articulated by Medard Gabel, former Executive Director of the World Game Institute, a UN-affiliated NGO. Gabel describes it this way:

> Regenerative development is characterized by a global and long-term perspective and approach that builds our capacity for qualitative growth. It values and needs input from all stakeholders; is transparent so that everyone can see how they win and what they might need to give up to gain a greater good; sees problems and needs as markets for social and economic entrepreneurs; and utilizes design that relies on doing more with less to accomplish its ends. It is focused on the vision of what is desired, not what is expedient…rather than reacting to what is thought possible given current limitations, regenerative development is in tune with nature, with what the world wants, and with the resources and technology that can take us there. (Gabel 2015, p.1)

Working therapeutically with individuals and groups can also support a shift in society at large. In the words of Thích Nhất Hạnh, a pioneer of Ecological Buddhism, "There is suffering, fear and anger inside of us, and when we take care of it, we are taking care of the world" (Hoggan 2016, p.195). As mental health practitioners, we can step up to become transformational leaders who contribute to the conversations about the important role that psychology plays in initiating change.

Mental health professionals and their clients as transformational leaders

In 2016 an interesting article appeared in the *New York Times*: "Why therapists should talk politics," by New York psychotherapist Richard Brouillette. In it, Brouillette affirms the following:

> It is inherently therapeutic to help a person understand the injustice of his predicament, reflect on the question of his own agency, and take whatever action he sees fit… Therapists need to consider such political interaction in the consulting room as inherent to the therapeutic process. Patients become motivated to change the world around them as a solution to what had become internal stressors. This is an experience of not just external but internal change, bringing

new confidence and a sense of engagement that becomes a part of the patient's character. (Brouillette 2016, p.1)

Leadership is about hope. Everyone who is awakening to climate change reality and is active in any part of the "Great Turning" is doing transformational work, and both mental health professionals and their clients carry the potential for moving into transformational leadership. Many of the concepts are already embedded in the nature of what we provide as therapists. While we remain client-centered, and rarely advise anyone about what they ought to do, we are nevertheless supporting valuable and positive change in both individual and social systems, which is the essence of transformational leadership (Kouzes and Posner 1999). We enhance our clients' motivation and effectiveness by understanding their strengths and challenges. We can help our clients align their behaviors to optimize their life goals.

The Pachamama Alliance, a non-profit global community committed to "creating a sustainable future that works for all" (Pachamama Alliance 2016, p.1) has adapted many of the core principles of transformational leadership into climate change work. As part of its "Game Changer Intensive" training, it articulates ten qualities of a "game changer," a transformational leader. The following principles are especially relevant to our work when we are assisting clients with climate-change-related issues:

1. *You understand that all life is connected.* You see the human family in all its diversity as an integral component in the whole web of creation.

2. *You stand for a sustainable, just, and fulfilling future.* You stand for and act from an informed vision that a sustainable, just, and fulfilling future for all beings is urgent, possible, and essential.

3. *You [assist clients to] inquire deeply.* You understand that the collective transformation of our society requires a completely new definition of what is possible in being human and requires that we inquire deeply into questions such as, "Who am I, really?" and "What is my relationship to the whole?"

4. *You [facilitate clients to] put forth a new story.* You are able to discern the cultural stories that perpetuate inequality and concentrate

power and privilege, and you live from...the paradigm for a just and sustainable future. (Pachamama Alliance 2016, p.1)

A worthy transformational leader in our field is not a therapist who creates followers, but rather one who encourages qualities of leadership to grow within their clients. As with any therapeutic shift, there are many factors that influence the scope and timing of change. The clinical artistry of how and when we support, empathize, interpret, and challenge remain within the domain of each person's theoretical approach and experience. But there has never been a more important time or a more vital role for therapists to include in the scope of their practice than this: a clinical awareness of the evolutionary transformation that is occurring right now.

Additional resources

Game Changer Intensive: A seven-week, online course through Pachamama Alliance: www.pachamama.org/engage/intensive

Hawken, P. (2007) *Blessed Unrest: How the Largest Social Movement in History is Restoring Grace, Justice and Beauty to the World.* New York, NY: Penguin Books.

Roszak, T. (2001) *The Voice of the Earth: An Exploration of Ecopsychology.* Grand Rapids, MI: Phanes Press.

Solnit, R. (2016) *Hope in the Dark: Untold Histories, Wild Possibilities.* Chicago, IL: Haymarket Books.

WORKSHEET
Transformational leadership

Self-inquiry: being a transformational leader

Buckminster Fuller asked, "If the success or failure of this planet and of human beings depended on how I am and what I do, how would I be? What would I do?"(Jedlicka 2010, p.190). Reflect on Pachamama's second quality of transformational leadership: "You stand for a sustainable, just and fulfilling future." Can you imagine three specific ways that this principle could manifest in your life?

1. _____

2. _____

3. _____

Coming home to yourself

Working with people who are suffering extreme loss can easily trigger our own feelings of distress. Self-care is an essential part of participating in any efforts in the field of climate change advocacy. Try this self-care approach, and feel free to modify it in any way that serves you:[3]

Set aside 15 minutes at the end of your workday when you can be free from interruptions. This practice can release the focus of your day and provide a way to reconnect with yourself.

Close your eyes and take three clearing breaths.

As you breathe in, infuse your body, heart, and mind with fresh oxygen, feeling and imagining it traveling from head to toe. When you exhale, release your focus on thoughts and invite your body to relax. Let your mind become aware of and follow the movements in your body of inhalation and exhalation—the rise and fall of your belly and the expansion and release of rib cage. Invite each clearing breath to be slow, full, and long.

Now let your breath settle into its own rhythm. Call into your awareness, one by one, the significant interactions of the day: clients, friends, and strangers. As each one appears, take a moment to honor the interaction and the person, and then with a breath of kindness, release them from your focus and send their energy back to them.

When they are all released, turn your awareness toward the direct experience of your own vitality and sense of wellbeing. Sense those qualities in your body. You may recognize your vitality as an image, a color or light, or a physical sensation. However you experience it, take the next five minutes to practice nourishing breaths.

When you breathe in, feel and imagine the oxygen from your breath strengthening your vitality. If you imagine it as a light, it may gradually shine brighter. If it is a color, it may shift and change. Simply breathe in, receiving nourishment; breathe out, simply rest. While the images may or may not change, the practice is to simply breathe in, receiving nourishment; breathe out, simply rest.

After five minutes, notice any changes, however subtle, in your body, mind, and emotions. Feel yourself present and grounded in your body, and when you are ready open your eyes. Take the next five minutes to move a little more slowly than you usually do, as you continue into your day or evening.

Chapter 4

Mindful Disaster Response

Perspectives from Ground Zero

While this book is primarily a resource for mental health professionals working in private practice or clinics, there is a growing need for psychological support to accompany on-site disaster relief efforts. Disaster mental health involves delivering services at ground zero, being a liaison to practical infrastructure aid, and employing a crisis intervention focus. This is a radically different therapeutic environment—often chaotic, with a lack of privacy, a team approach, no defined appointment times, and working with people who might not seek out therapeutic support in a more traditional setting. Disaster mental health is a therapeutic specialization with diverse approaches and theoretical orientations, and this chapter will distill its essential clinical themes and provide resources for pursuing more in-depth training. For mental health professionals with some systems savvy, good self-care, openhearted empathetic listening, and a desire to be of service at times of high need, this can be a rewarding way to offer your skills, either as a volunteer or by committing to a new professional specialization.

Therapy without walls

According to the Federal Emergency Management Agency (FEMA), a major disaster is defined as "any natural catastrophe, or regardless of cause, any fire, flood, or explosion that causes damage of sufficient severity and magnitude to warrant assistance supplementing State, local, and disaster relief organization efforts to alleviate damage, loss, hardship, or suffering" (FEMA 1995, p.1). It is easy to see in this core definition of disaster relief how emotional care is an essential part of the overall effort. Research documents that immediate psychosocial support following a disaster consistently buffers against prolonged stress and trauma (Norris, *et al.* 2002).

Hands-on therapeutic work with communities is a complex undertaking, and the emotional and social wellbeing of a community must be understood and approached with respect for its historical and cultural identities (Landau 2007; Walsh 2007). The American Family Therapy Academy (AFTA) Action Research Team (AART) studied best practices for effectively promoting community resilience in the face of a catastrophe, and they emphasize the importance of a collaborative model. Their recommendations are built on three principles.

1. Honor the work of local community groups.

2. Honor the language, knowledge, goals, and intentions of community members when formulating the project, carrying out the project, and documenting the project.

3. Follow the wishes of community members when reporting on any work done, that is, accounts to local newspapers, papers at conferences, or published papers.

(Bava et al. 2010, p.549)

Whenever possible, it is tremendously helpful to empower local community groups with self-aware and conscious leadership and membership that are resilient and resourceful in an emergency. When the voice of the community is invalidated or minimized by relief groups, or social justice perspectives are not taken into account, it can actually *increase* long-term post-trauma distress (Pennebaker and Harber 1993). To promote mutual decision-making from the outset, it is recommended that service providers obtain a community invitation, although frequently there are obstacles to obtaining a definitive authorization. At the scene of large-scale disasters, there are usually teams from multiple relief organizations, and it can be challenging to coordinate services. While our role is mental health support, we are part of a collaborative effort to provide a comprehensive range of services, because "empowerment without resources is counterproductive and demoralizing" (Hobfoll *et al.* 2007, p.295).

DISASTER RELIEF GROUPS WITHIN THE THERAPEUTIC COMMUNITY

Because of the importance of community cohesiveness, it can be a powerful initiative to either join or create a disaster response mental health team in your own area, where the unique culture and local resources of the community are already known. You can check with the county or regional chapter of your professional mental health association to learn what may already be in place or to host a new committee and training program. If you are interested in serving on national or international teams, there are many established disaster mental health groups you can join that have experience and finesse in navigating the complexities of supporting diverse communities.

Many of the specific therapeutic treatment approaches known to be effective with trauma—such as Eye Movement Desensitization and Reprocessing (EMDR) and Somatic Experiencing—have organized volunteer disaster relief trainings and teams comprised of mental health professionals. By joining the group that best suits your therapeutic training, you would find built-in expertise, professional support, and logistical orientation. Here are a few of the active, well-established organizations that utilize mental health professionals in disaster relief work.

American Red Cross

The American Red Cross collaborates with local professional mental health association chapters, and can provide resources for basic training and orientation. Volunteering with the Red Cross Disaster Mental Health (DMH) team includes providing assessment, triage, and crisis intervention for community members impacted by disaster. Emotional support can also include counseling other Red Cross workers who are experiencing the stress of a disaster. Red Cross DMH workers must have an active license to practice independently in the state where they live. The teams can include clinical social workers, licensed marriage and family therapists, professional counselors, psychiatric nurses, psychiatrists, psychologists, and school counselors. You can find more information at redcross.org.

Guided imagery/mind–body tools
Guided imagery is well documented as an effective treatment for post-traumatic stress disorder, and it is recommended by the U.S. Veterans Administration. The Center for Mind-Body Medicine, founded by James Gordon, M.D., uses guided imagery along with other mind–body approaches, including meditation, biofeedback, and creative self-expression. Gordon's team has brought his protocol to numerous sites worldwide, including Haiti, Gaza, New Orleans, and Kosovo, to heal trauma and help build resilient communities. For more information, visit cmbm.org.

Somatic Experiencing
Dr. Peter Levine, founder of Somatic Experiencing, teaches clinical tools to assess and resolve stress responses, guiding clients to release suppressed emotions and increase their capacity to tolerate trauma-based physical sensations. The organization has recently added a curriculum specific to disaster response, and it has successfully taken this work into a variety of locations including Haiti, the Congo, and post-tsunami Japan. More information can be found at traumahealing.org.

Eye Movement Desensitization and Reprocessing (EMDR)
The EMDR Humanitarian Assistance Program (HAP) has provided recovery assistance as part of local emergency response teams in communities impacted by natural disasters, including Hurricanes Katrina and Sandy, the 2004 tsunami in Thailand, and the tornadoes in Joplin, Missouri, and Tuscaloosa, Alabama. If you are already trained in EMDR bilateral trauma treatment, you can get additional support and disaster mental health training from its HAP Trauma Recovery Network. Its website is emdrhap.org.

Expressive arts therapy
Community Healing through Art (CHART) is a non-profit coalition of professional artists, art therapists, and expressive arts facilitators that was founded in 2005 following the South Asian earthquake and tsunami. They provide disaster training and orientation and often partner with universities and service organizations. Their teams have worked in New Orleans, Thailand, India, Sri Lanka, South Africa, Bahamas, Haiti, New Zealand, and Japan. Expressive arts help clients transform their internal experience into an external form, which provides greater clarity, integration, and relief. It also offers a non-verbal outlet that can then

support other forms of therapeutic processing. You can find out more at this site: communitieshealingthroughart.tumblr.com.

Mindful Disaster Mental Health

Whether or not you choose to participate in community-based Disaster Mental Health (DMH), clinical issues related to climate psychology will likely show up in your practice. Whatever therapeutic theories and modalities comprise your approach, mindfulness is a valuable addition to the work of building resiliency and personal empowerment in the face of climate change, and it can be easily integrated into most clinical styles.

Mindfulness involves bringing awareness to thoughts, feelings, and sensations in the present moment with an attitude of acceptance and curiosity. It cultivates a willingness to experience a full range of feelings and thoughts without self-criticism or filters. While mindfulness is historically rooted in Buddhism, it is currently a widespread practice in the West that finds numerous applications in mainstream medicine, education, business, and psychology.

Mindfulness decreases symptoms of anxiety and depression (Kabat-Zinn *et al.* 1992; Siegel 2002) and is increasingly being applied in the treatment of post-traumatic stress disorder (Vujanovic *et al.* 2009). Mindfulness can mitigate physiological arousal and foster emotional regulation (Baer 2003; Shapiro 1982).

FUNCTIONAL TREMBLING

Recent research has emphasized that trauma is held in the nervous system, and some clients find it initially too overwhelming to bring mindful attention to their physical sensations. For these individuals, it can be very helpful to interweave body-based release therapies like Bioenergetics, SomatoEmotional Release, Hakomi, Tension and Trauma Releasing (TRE), EMDR, Emotional Freedom Technique (EFT), or walking meditation prior to beginning more traditional silent mindfulness practices.

Neurogenic tremors—trembling or shivering—are the body's natural response to stress and trauma and a sign of the system's efforts to restore normal function (Payne, Levine, and Crane-Godreau 2015). We see it in everyday experiences: "I was terrified and my hands were shaking," "My legs were shaking when it was time to walk on stage," "I was so upset that my jaw was quivering." The shaking is a restorative mechanism that releases us from the stress-induced "freeze response," and Levine (1997) proposes that we can intentionally mirror the adaptation of wild animals as they "shake out" the stress and become fully functional again.

While these trauma-informed treatments involve special training and prescribe specific protocols, the following is a simple practice that can get the energy moving and releasing throughout the body, and is a great way to take a break during group processing. It also adds a playful levity that can be very beneficial.

Dog Remedy

Can you recall the way a wet dog dries itself off with a progressive shimmy-shake that starts with the head and travels to the tail, water drops spraying in a cascading halo? We can use this image to "shake off" some of our own stress. This exercise can be done with an individual or in a group of any size. Demonstrate the exercise as you describe it, emphasizing that there is no "right way" to do the movement: the important part is the shaking itself. While this is a gentle movement practice, remind participants to move safely and respect their body's limitations.

Stand with your feet shoulder-distance apart to create a solid base. Begin gently shaking just your head—side to side, up and down. Take about ten seconds with the head and with each area of the body. Now let your head rest, but keep the shaking going in your shoulders. After about ten seconds, let the shaking travel into your arms and hands, as if you were flicking water off your fingers. Let the shaking move to your torso and hips, bringing as much mobility as possible to the ribcage and pelvis. The final segment is to let the shaking travel down each leg one at a time, alternating lifting each foot off the floor and flicking "water" from the toes. If balance is a concern, a chair back can be used for stability when standing on one foot, or both feet can remain on the floor, with alternating heel taps.

Repeat the "dog remedy" progression about six times, increasing the speed that the shaking progresses through the body until the final one is one quick, shimmering flow.

Within climate psychology work, assisting clients to practice mindfulness and other reflective practices can help them increase self-compassion, access their inherent strengths, increase their capacity to tolerate intense experiences, and cultivate present-moment awareness rather than living in flashbacks or numbing out. These skills are profoundly useful with any degree of climate-induced stress. Additional practices that teach these skills are included throughout this chapter and the book.

WINDOW OF TOLERANCE

An important concept in trauma-focused treatment is the "window of tolerance," a term coined by Dan Siegel (2012). It refers to an optimal range of emotional and physiological arousal within which we can thrive and function most effectively. Many factors influence our range of tolerance, including our temperament, attachment style, previous losses and traumas, and the degree to which we are presently depleted by fatigue and hunger. Too much distress prompts our nervous system to enter the stress response, pushing us into hyperarousal. This can manifest as irritation, rage, intrusive images, acting out, and other strong emotions, and we typically lack the capacity to regulate these experiences. For those more prone to dissociate, high stress may cause withdrawal, a shutting-down into a state of hypoarousal, which likewise interferes with our ability to make clear decisions and engage with our circumstances in a functional manner. The prefrontal cortex, which helps modulate our emotions, shuts down in both of these extreme reaction states. The limbic system and brain stem, home of our more primitive emotional reactivity, remains engaged, severely compromising our ability to process our experience successfully (Post *et al.* 1997).

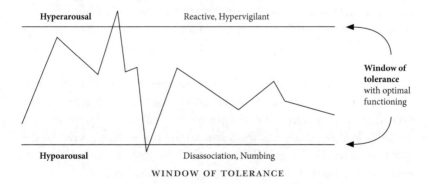

WINDOW OF TOLERANCE

Trauma creates a narrowing of the window of tolerance (Siegel 2012), and mindfulness can widen it through experiences of self-regulation and self-soothing that build resiliency. With mindful awareness of body sensations, thoughts, and emotions, clients who are experiencing climate-provoked stress acquire the ability to recognize when they are nearing the edge of their tolerance and begin practices that will help them remain within their optimal response zone. With mindfulness, adaptability and flexibility are enhanced.

As with all the approaches used in climate psychology work, mindfulness is not simply about coping. Initially, we must reclaim the resources and internal stability in order to be present enough simply to function. Mindfulness also takes us to a deeper sense of who we are, so that we can emerge from chaos with a greater connection to our humanity and participate more fully in evolutionary transformation. Jakusho Kwong-roshi, Abbot of the Sonoma Mountain Zen Center, adds that "original mindfulness [is the] actualization of humanity's inherent basic goodness" (Rappaport 2014, p.13). Mindfulness can open our hearts and minds so that we see each other more kindly and cultivate the qualities that prepare us for action rooted in clarity and calmness. This kind of grounded presence is not necessarily about heroic acts: being fully present to simple things, in small actions, can be tremendously healing and powerful.

Mindfulness is ultimately practical. Christiana Figueres, the former Executive Secretary of the United Nations Framework Convention on Climate Change, has been involved in climate change negotiations since 1995. She led the climate negotiations at COP21 in Paris in 2015, where 196 countries assembled to obtain a global agreement—amidst significant resistance—to reduce the carbon emissions that are creating runaway climate change. Some describe her job as near-impossible, but when we learn that she has this framed quote hung above her desk, we get a sense of her resilient spirit: "Impossible is not a fact, it is an attitude" (Kolbert 2015, p.1).

Figueres credits Thích Nhất Hạnh, a Zen Buddhist monk, with assisting her to cultivate the compassion, wisdom, and strength she needed to negotiate the climate agreements that were forged over two intensive weeks with leaders from around the world. Hạnh is one of the best-known teachers of mindfulness in the West and has himself been an environmental activist for more than 20 years (Confino 2016).

Three stages of climate disaster recovery

As with the model of the stages of grief, a disaster recovery model must have a flexible structure that encompasses many variables in order to address a diverse range of individuals and communities. The Department of Veterans Affairs, along with the National Center for Post-Traumatic Stress Disorder, created a guidebook of disaster mental health services that delineates three phases of disaster recovery. These stages are valuable to keep in mind, whether you are providing services on-site or working with individuals and families who come to your office.

EMERGENCY STAGE: DURING AND IMMEDIATELY FOLLOWING A DISASTER

The survivors you meet may have just lost the world that was known to them: time is fractured, place is unfamiliar and disorienting, people are emotionally stunned and numb. There is collective trauma as an entire area is suffering extreme loss. Your professional clarity of mind and kind presence fills in for the individuals' usual capacities that have temporarily shut down due to shock. You will want to determine whether basic needs are taken care of, including safety, shelter, food, water, transportation, and sanitation. Be sure that individuals are able to connect to supportive people who they can reach out to at any time, day or night. Assist their movement away from the areas of destruction and toward safety, loved ones, and support.

There will likely be some members of the community who are eager to help and who are capable of joining the support structure. One way they can assist is by providing information and access to resources that only local residents would know about. Helping can be part of disaster victims' own recovery, and it is essential to support and empower their role within appropriate parameters, working with them in a team and strengthening their role in the community.

It is important to normalize all feelings and experiences, including lack of feeling. Because mental health professionals typically provide services that help alleviate distress, it can be tempting to offer reassurance about the disaster recovery when, in reality, there remain many unknowns. Instead, it is more therapeutic to address immediate needs, affirm experiences compassionately, and offer simple tools for self-soothing while cultivating present-moment awareness. Here is a simple practice that can be very useful in the early stages of disaster recovery. It can be taught individually or in a group setting.

Mindful bilateral tapping
Originally called the Butterfly Hug, the bilateral tapping technique was developed in 1998 by EMDR therapist Lucina Artigas when she traveled to Acapulco, Mexico, to assist in disaster recovery after Hurricane Pauline (Jarero, Artigas, and Montero 2008). The Butterfly Hug is a simple, bilateral stimulation method that emerged spontaneously during work with large groups in the disaster setting. Bilateral tapping promotes emotional regulation for both children and adults, although you may want to simplify the language for kids. The version presented here is modified from the original protocol, and blends the Bilateral Tapping Technique with mindfulness practice.[1]

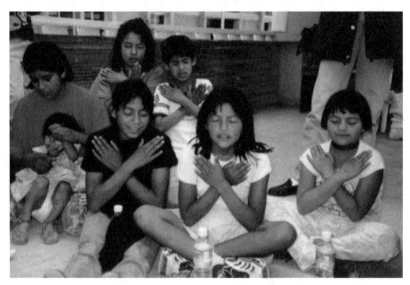

BUTTERFLY HUG TECHNIQUE, MEXICO CITY
IN RESPONSE TO A FIRE

MINDFUL BILATERAL TAPPING PRACTICE

Sit or stand comfortably upright, and take a moment to feel the natural weight of your feet resting solidly on the ground if you are standing or the sensations of the chair supporting your body if you are sitting. Let your eyes have a soft focus. Take three conscious breaths while you pay attention to the soft sensations of support.

(The therapist demonstrates while offering instructions.)

Now cross your arms over your chest, with each hand resting just below the collarbones, fingers pointing upward toward the neck (not toward the arms), and your elbows resting against your torso. Acknowledge whatever you are feeling, and state it silently to yourself:

This is a moment of… (use the most accurate word) *suffering, struggle, sadness, fear, upset, distress, pain, loss, etc.*

Notice whatever feelings and sensations accompany your statement. Staying aware of the feelings and sensations, now begin to alternately tap each shoulder with the palms of your hands, letting the feelings and any accompanying images just pass through your awareness like you are watching a movie, or a train going by.

After about three minutes, relax your arms by your sides and take three more conscious breaths, once again returning your attention to the sensations of support.

Cross your arms over your chest one more time, now saying silently to yourself: *I offer myself the* (use the most accurate word) *patience, kindness, strength, rest, compassion, etc. I need right now.*

Repeat this phrase for three minutes with the alternate hand tapping. Without trying to make anything in particular happen, allow any soothing images or feelings that spontaneously arise to become part of your experience.

Relax your arms by your sides and bring this practice to a close with three conscious breaths, aware once again of the sensations of support.

The practice can be done several times throughout each day.

EARLY POST-IMPACT: THE DAY AFTER THROUGH 12 WEEKS

During this early post-event period, there will continue to be practical needs that need to be addressed in tandem with emotional care. Social relationships will be strained, with families whose homes have been severely damaged or destroyed often relocating multiple times before settling again more permanently. Sometimes family members are separated from one another and live scattered among relatives. Kids may be adjusting to new, temporary schools (Tapsell and Tunstall 2008).

Inquire whether the people you are seeing take prescription medications and if they have access to them, including psychotropic stabilizers. Individuals with addiction are at risk of relapse due to the high degree of stress and disruption to their established support. Connect them as soon as possible to resources that can address medical needs.

Adrenaline and exhaustion levels are liable to be high, and it remains important to support the re-establishment of basic routines including rest, sleep, and regular meals. It is very helpful to affirm the strength-based behaviors you observe with words like, "It's great the way you're taking care of...[yourself, your family, your neighbor]."

As the days and weeks progress, mental health care begins to shift from impromptu sessions to more structured and coordinated services. This is a time for debriefing and defusing, but it is also important to build internal resiliency and mindful resourcefulness at the same time, so that any therapeutic dialogue that includes a recall of recent events is not re-traumatizing.

The resiliency practice "Remembered Strength" helps reconnect individuals with inherent qualities that have helped them cope successfully with difficult times in the past and to evoke those strengths in the current situation. The type of strength to be remembered is determined by the client; the range is broad and can include resilient qualities like patience, assertiveness, courage, kindness, trust, and calm. This kind of remembering is much more holistic than simply recalling a visual memory. The practice evokes a remembered felt-sense of the qualities, reconnecting to the somatic and emotional experience. It is a visceral knowing, a body-based confidence. These kinds of practices may be new to some individuals or communities; and to even pause and reflect for a short time may seem counterproductive given the urgency and scope of what needs to be accomplished. It is helpful to offer simple, research-based education and a practical rationale, which can include citing the way that these tools increase energy and alertness, improve sleep, and assist with clarity in decision-making.

Depending on the client's readiness, this practice can be done in stages, with a session devoted just to the breath practice, and then progressive relaxation can be added in a second meeting before combining it with the quality retrieval process.

REMEMBERED STRENGTH

Find the quietest, most private setting available, aiming for at least 30 minutes of undisturbed time.

Through conversation, help the client identify one quality they wish they could experience in their present situation, such as patience, strength, or courage. Have them describe a time in the past when they had a strong experience of that quality. Ask them if they would be willing to explore the possibility of reconnecting with their chosen quality though a relaxation exercise. If they agree, let them know that they can open their eyes at any time and that you will be asking them to speak aloud during their relaxation experience. Answer any questions they have about the process before beginning.

Invite them to get as comfortable as possible, and either close their eyes or maintain a soft downward gaze. Guide them through a brief progressive relaxation (see the Appendix for a complete script).

Therapist: *Now allow your mind to drift back in time, three months...six months...to...*(refer to the experience of strength they selected. Example: "That time at the baseball field when you felt such courage when helping your injured son."). *As your memory comes fully alive, describe aloud what you're aware of.*

Help the client enliven their memory by inquiring about the colors, textures, sounds, and smells from that time and place. *Now find that feeling of...*(their chosen quality*) and step into that experience again. Notice how the* (quality) *feels in your body, your mind, and your emotions.* (Pause, allowing time for them to really reconnect to the experience.) *Keeping your eyes closed, describe aloud what you're noticing now.* (If they can somatically recall the feeling, allow extra time for them to be present in their experience. If they need assistance, you can ask *What would help you feel more* (the quality) *right now, knowing that many things are possible in this relaxed state?* If they describe a suggestion, help guide them into that experience.)

Stay connected to the (quality), *feeling it once more in your body, mind, and heart. Allow the image of the* (memory) *to fade, but continue to feel the* (quality), *slowing bringing it back with you to the present moment, into this place and time.*

Notice again the (quality) *while you feel once more the chair you are sitting in...hear the sounds in this room... Feel the* (quality) *as you notice the rise and fall of your breath, and the temperature of the air. Still remaining connected to your* (quality), *when you're ready gently open your eyes.*

Take time to let the client describe their experiences. Good questions to ask include the following.

- How are you feeling now?

- Were there any surprises?

- What is your "take-away" from this experience?

Rather than interpreting their experience, support the client in cultivating and reconnecting with their resilient quality. It can be useful for them to draw or write about their experience as a way to continue integrating it. Returning to the picture or writing is also a touchstone that can support their ongoing connection to the desired quality.

When individuals and communities experience emotional trauma, they naturally talk and think about it. If they continue thinking about the event but are unable to process the experience with others, they are at increased risk for both psychological and health issues (Pennebaker and Harber 1993). Writer James Baldwin reminds us, "Not everything that is faced can be changed, but nothing can be changed until it is faced" (Baldwin 2011, p.42). It is useful to toggle back and forth between supporting their present-moment mindfulness and inner resiliency and talking about all their experiences and feelings, which may include fear, helplessness, and loss. You can invoke brief "mindful moments" that can include parts of the previous exercises, such as noticing the sensations of their feet, three conscious breaths, or brief bilateral tapping.

There are two standard protocols in disaster mental health treatment at this early post-event stage: defusing and debriefing.

Defusing: one-on-one

Bruce Young and Julian Ford with the National Center for Post-Traumatic Stress Disorder developed a six-step process to be used on-site: make contact, assess, gather facts, inquire about thoughts, inquire about feelings, and support, reassure, and provide information (Young, et al. 1998). This may sound like a condensed version of a basic psychotherapeutic treatment plan, but it is distinctly different when performed at a disaster site. In a private practice, "making contact" means building rapport over time, performing an intake, and establishing a therapeutic contract. At ground zero, making contact begins with casual socializing—perhaps you are standing in a food line and strike up an informal conversation: "Can I get you some water or tea?" During this kind of casual contact, an assessment can occur as you track the concerns they express and the person's apparent physical tension, emotional lability, mental clarity and cohesiveness, etc. You can introduce your role and offer to help them gain information or to assist with other needs they have revealed.

If possible, seek a more private space, which may simply be an unoccupied corner of a large tent or community room. To continue the debriefing, you can begin to inquire into thoughts and feelings.

- What ran through your mind when the disaster happened?

- What is the hardest part about the event?

- Is there anything anyone said to you that stands out in your memory?

- What thoughts will you carry with you?

- What has helped you cope so far?

(Young et al. 1998, pp.41–42)

When the survivors regain access to their damaged homes and community, there is a strong desire to sift through debris for practical, valuable, and sentimental objects. Many feelings are likely to arise as items are either retrieved or never recovered: relief at finding a driver's license, despair over a broken guitar, and desperation when looking for a wedding ring. There are often distorted thoughts as the mind grapples to make sense of what happened: "If only I had followed my instincts, I could have saved my dog," "I'll never be happy again," "I shouldn't be so selfish—others have it worse off than me." If you have additional training in methods like EMDR, EFT, or Somatic Experiencing, it can be valuable to add these treatments, following the clinical protocols for these methods.

Debriefing: group
Critical Incident Stress Debriefing (CISD) was developed in 1974 by Jeffrey Mitchell, Ph.D., Clinical Professor of Emergency Health Services at the University of Maryland. It is a psycho-educational group process designed to normalize group members' reactions to a critical incident and facilitate their recovery (Mitchell 1983). It was originally designed for first responders—paramedics, police officers, firefighters—who experienced intense distress through exposure to horrific accidents and disasters. CISD is now used with a variety of populations, though the traditional method requires a homogeneous group of about 20 people with the same level of exposure to the experience and who are psychologically ready to engage. CISD can be conducted anywhere from 24 hours to several weeks following the disaster. While it used to be a standard treatment protocol, it is now used more sporadically. You would only use CISD if it is offered in the impacted area and you have had the training.

While traditional CISD follows a strict protocol, many of its key elements of facilitated storytelling along with teaching stress-management tools have been modified and used with a variety of populations. Following Hurricane Iniki in 1992 in Hawaii, one of the most costly natural disasters in the United States' history at the time, research was conducted using a variation of group debriefing. It focused on venting and normalizing feelings along with education about psychological reactions to the disaster. This study was randomized with two groups who experienced the hurricane. Those who participated in the debriefing had a substantial reduction in their hurricane-related distress and a significant decrease in symptoms (Chemtob *et al.* 1997).

RESTORATION STAGE: THREE MONTHS, ONGOING...

Depending on the scope and intensity of the disaster, it can take months to years for infrastructure to be rebuilt and the psychological impact to diminish. The survivor's sense of time will be punctuated by anniversaries of the event, and particular places will evoke harsh memories.

As the weeks and months progress, brief glimpses of new possibilities begin to emerge through the dark images of chaos. Time grows ripe with the potential for rebuilding a cohesive community infrastructure and learning to invoke resilient psychological perspectives. As mental health professionals, we can encourage the capacity to reflect deeply on the meaning of what has occurred and what is now possible. We can highlight and support the natural moments of grace, courage, and strength that spontaneously begin to arise within the community.

The need to rebuild offers the opportunity to consider a more ecoharmonious system that involves a renewed connection to nature, life, people, and the planet. There is an opening to plunge the depths of the geography of our own human soul, bringing to the surface a map for the kind of world we can sense is possible after we release cynicism and despair. On some level, we all know that the human interface with the world can be more kind and beautiful, and these aspirations can begin to be actualized as new internal and external foundations are built.

Building community

The type of living environment impacted by a climate change crisis—suburban, rural, or urban—will have a strong influence on the kind of structured group communication that can most easily take shape. One rural mountain community held town meetings every two weeks for years following a major flood, and virtually every resident was a consistent and eager participant. In larger urban areas people tend to be more disconnected from each other, and groups will often form in neighborhoods, schools, churches, and settings where people already gather for established reasons. Regardless of the setting, telling and listening to stories that contain each person's insights, talents, concerns, hopes, and creativity is a key component in building community.

Continuing to heal emotions while building infrastructure can be challenging as diverse perspectives arise. Structured processes can support the capacity to think and converse more deeply, while also fostering trust and reducing barriers to cooperation. Specific group process structures can evoke a sense of possibility and provide tools for reducing contentiousness and the risk of becoming mired in conflict.

Some of the most effective group forms I have found are those that blend the best of modern group process with indigenous structures for intentional conversation. The broad term is a wisdom or sacred circle, and there are many models, such as "Council" and "World Café," that have been successful in building community in settings as diverse as peace-building in Rwanda, working with refugees, facilitating conversations between government officials and farmers in Mexico, and building trust among inmates in prison systems.

While these are not therapy groups, and they often are facilitated by trained volunteers, your foundation in good communication skills will be a real asset. The basic guidelines for these kinds of gatherings include a method for hosting collaborative dialogues. Here is the typical format.

- The group sits in a circle with a defined center, which can be created collectively with meaningful objects or flowers placed by each participant, or art materials to use as part of the process.

- A facilitator/witness serves as the timekeeper and explains the guidelines. While no one is required to speak or participate in any exercise, everyone is encouraged to participate. For ongoing meetings, the role of facilitator can rotate among group members.

- Guidelines include creating safety with confidentiality, sharing personal experiences without giving advice to other members, and using "I statements." Members can be reminded that the intention is to honor and respect each person in the circle and to listen with a spirit of curiosity.

- The number of participants is generally no more than 12 in a circle. For a large community group, smaller circles can be formed, with time at the end for each circle to summarize for the whole group the themes that arose. Circles generally last one-and-a-half to two hours, and the timeline should be determined in advance.

- There is usually a grounding or centering meditation to open the group. This helps set the tone for a deeper dialogue. It could be as simple as a minute of silence or a more structured guided meditation using breath work, body scanning, and images relevant to the theme. The opening could also take the form of a simple ritual, such as lighting a candle or reading a poem.

- A question or theme relevant to the stage of disaster recovery can focus the dialogue in the circle. Examples include: What draws us together? How can we carry the spirit of this meeting back into our community? How can I remain open to hope? How can I help others and take care of myself too? What is my vision for our changing community and world?

- Use a "talking piece." This can be any object that can be easily held in one hand. Only the person holding the talking piece can speak. This prevents cross-talk and interruptions and initiates a pause between speakers for deeper reflection as the piece is placed back in the center.

- Members are encouraged to listen for key connections between diverse viewpoints, insights, patterns, and underlying questions or assumptions.

- It is very useful to allow time for drawing or writing in silence. This can be done at the beginning when the theme is presented or following the circle dialogue. This allows for nonverbal processing and other ways to share.

- Bring the circle to closure, respecting the agreed upon timeline. Closing can take many forms, but it needs to be intentional and in keeping with the feel of the gathering. Examples include each person briefly stating what they will take away from the collective dialogue. It could end with a moment of silence or each person saying one word that reflects how they are feeling.

- If the circle is part of a larger community meeting, be sure to allow time for each circle to let a spokesperson summarize and share themes with the larger group (Brown and Isaacs 2005; Garfield, Spring, and Cahill 1998; Seide 2016; Zimmerman and Coyle 2009).

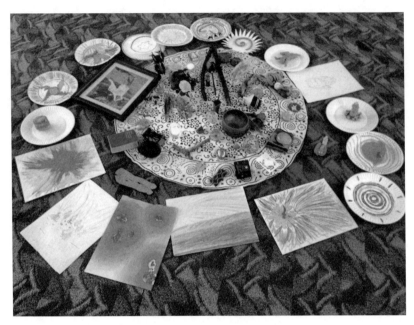

CENTER FOR COUNCIL

Visioning possibility

Whether we are prompted by a natural disaster or we have a preventative ecological focus, we can use any opportunity to open our imaginations in a new way. We may be treading on ground that shifts between hope and despair, and it requires a nimble and attentive heart and creative frame of mind to cultivate balance and find inspiration to build a healthier lifestyle. The Bulgarian writer Maria Popova stated, "Critical thinking without hope is cynicism. Hope without critical thinking is naïveté" (Popova 2015, p.1)—and it is stretching ourselves to hold these polarities that can, perhaps surprisingly, provide a focused direction. Embracing an expanded perspective shapes us: it keeps our feet on the ground, our minds focused on potential, and our hearts open to connection. Pema Chödrön, Director of Buddhist Gampo Abbey describes it this way:

> Life is glorious, but life is also wretched. It is both. Appreciating the gloriousness inspires us, encourages us, cheers us up, gives us a bigger perspective, energizes us. We feel connected... On the other hand, wretchedness—life's painful aspect—softens us up considerably. Knowing pain is a very important ingredient of being there for

another person. When you are feeling a lot of grief, you can look right into somebody's eyes because you feel you haven't got anything to lose—you're just there. The wretchedness humbles us and softens us, but if we were only wretched, we would all just go down the tubes… Gloriousness and wretchedness need each other. One inspires us, the other softens us. They go together. (Chödrön 2001, p.178)

Mindfulness cultivated within climate psychology can produce a tensile strength, kind and fierce commitment, focused openness, rooted expansiveness, and emotional intelligence in the midst of working with intense emotions. As mental health professionals, we bring relational skills. As we connect through compassionate listening, speaking, and action, these qualities can catch hold and ignite other hearts in a transforming world.

Additional resources

Follette, V., Briere, J., Rozelle, D., Hopper, J., and Rome, D. (eds) (2015) *Mindfulness-Oriented Interventions for Trauma: Integrating Contemplative Practices*. New York, NY: Guilford Press.

Garfield, C., Spring, C., and Cahill, S. (1998) *Wisdom Circles: A Guide to Discovery and Community Building in Small Groups*. New York, NY: Hyperion.

Graham, L. (2013) *Bouncing Back: Rewiring Your Brain for Maximum Resilience and Well-Being*. Novato, CA: New World Library.

Rendon, J. (2015) *Upside: The New Science of Post-Traumatic Growth*. New York, NY: Simon and Schuster.

WORKSHEET
Resiliency practices

What experiences have revealed to you your potentials and strengths? It could be as simple as learning that you can speak up for yourself in a challenging situation, make a significant life change, or achieve a goal. You could repeat the Remembered Strength practice with a different memory or write about another pivotal experience now.

While there are many practices to help us reconnect with our soothing and strengthening qualities during a difficult time, it is important to not try to "hurry up and feel better." Recovery has its own organic timing, and trusting your personal timeline is essential. This practice helps us be warm and caring toward ourselves and supports kind patience. Read through the instructions, and then try it with your eyes closed.

Remember and imagine as many of the moments of goodness and kindness that you have experienced in your life as you can. They may have come from family, friends, pets, strangers, spiritual guides, surprising opportunities. Imagine all that kindness like beams of loving light that can travel over continents and from the past into this moment. Let the warmth of these beams of goodness gather as a circle around you and shine directly on you. You may want to place one hand over your heart. When you inhale, receive the kindness and let it fill your body, heart, and mind. Really welcome it in. When you exhale, let that goodness find its home in you, abiding in every cell.

Do this practice for as long as you like, and for a minimum of five minutes, and do it as often as you like.

Chapter 5

Long-Term and Complex Clinical Themes

A sense of "home," of belonging, is one of the most powerful psychological needs in our human experience. Belonging often includes a place that has been built from a blend of connections, memories, history, hopes, and dreams. With climate change, a rupture with our bonds of place may begin, triggering an emotional response to changes in familiar landscapes. When you have that unsettling feeling that the natural environment right under your feet is changing for the worse, you are experiencing solastalgia. Coined by Glenn Albrecht, a faculty member in the Department of Sustainability at Murdoch University in Australia, the term is a blend of the words "solace" and "nostalgia" that captures our sense of distress. If we delve even deeper, we find that the Latin roots are a combination of "comfort" and "pain." Solastalgia means being homesick even when you have not left home (Aldern 2016).

In the previous chapter, we saw how anxiety and depression are aroused by severe environmental disasters created by our changing climate. We will now explore some of the more ongoing and subtle yet remarkably powerful psychological impacts of climate change, and offer clinical exercises to increase resilience.

Solastalgia

Deep connections are adaptive, like the enduring emotional bond that forms between an infant and caregiver articulated in attachment theory (Ainsworth 1973; Bowlby 1983). Similarly, place attachment is multifaceted and is defined by the emotional bond between a person and their environment that comprises our thoughts and feelings evoked by a place (Schroeder 1991). Robert Gifford, an environmental psychologist, finds great hope in that fact that, "Humans display an unwavering attachment to their place of dwelling" (Darabi 2015). It is this love of place that can spur people to take action—to take care of an environment they love in the same way they would fight to defend their family. Peter von Tiesenhausen's story is an inspiring example of one man's love of place and his remarkable success at defending his home.

Peter lives on 80-acre farm in Demmitt, Alberta, inherited from his parents. The land sits atop a deep basin of natural gas that the oil industry has been vigorously attempting to access since it was discovered in the 1970s. There are eminent domain issues at stake: the oil companies want to tap the underground fuel and run a natural gas pipeline across Peter's land. Peter works on the farm as a painter and sculptor. It is hard to imagine a happy outcome of an artist versus Big Oil battle, but so far Peter has retained the upper hand.

He has built a number of outdoor sculptures created specifically for the contours of the land. After brainstorming with a friend, he came up with the idea of registering his entire property as a work of art, claiming copyright over the land itself. He has been successful on multiple occasions, defending this earth art against the legal demands of powerful corporate interests. He also learned how to play their game, and began charging the oil companies $500 an hour for meetings with him. Between the long legal battle and the publicity it has engendered, the energy companies have backed off (Keefe 2014).

Clearly, Peter's strategy is very specific to the particular person and place, but it is an excellent example of how to put our imaginations to work and find success using whatever resources we can. It is a hopeful story in the "David and Goliath" proportions, and a great reminder to think creatively, especially when the odds are stacked against us.

We build resiliency in the face of solastalgia when we take care of and defend what matters most, including our environmental home. In our clinical practice, a client experiencing climate distress may not realize the ways in which action can facilitate psychological ease. We can help our clients explore how they can experience agency through greening and protecting their community—whether legislatively, creatively, or educationally.

Moral injury

"Moral injury" is a term used among veterans with war trauma that originated in the writings of Vietnam War veteran Camillo Bica (Brock and Lettini 2013), but it also has relevance for the suffering generated by the consequences of climate change. The U.S. Department of Veteran Affairs defines moral injury as, "An act of transgression, which shatters moral and ethical expectations that are rooted in religious or spiritual beliefs, or culture-based, organizational, and group-based rules about fairness, the value of life, and so forth" (Maguen and Litz 2015, p.1). If throughout Brock and Lettini's (2013) book *Soul Repair: Recovering from Moral Injury after War* you replaced the word "war" with "climate change," while there are obvious differences, many of the underlying themes would hold up remarkably well.

As the traumatic symptoms of a climate-related event subside, and time allows for a coherent narrative to emerge that describes the larger forces that contributed to the disaster, moral questions can arise: "How did our leaders let this happen? Who can I trust? In what ways am I complicit with an unethical system? Are we living in a moral and reasonable world?" Even if we made decisions that seemed right at the time, based on information we had at hand, as we look back at the unintended consequences we can move into shame and question our personal moral integrity.

As we have noted, there are many social justice issues interwoven into climate change that raise incisive moral questions. "Climate justice" is a term now being used to bring ethical and socially mediated perspectives—like including civic equality and human rights—into climate change discussions, rather than emphasizing just the environmental factors. A fundamental proposition of climate justice is that those who are least responsible for climate change suffer the most severe consequences (Skelton and Miller 2016). Pope Francis emphasized this in his Encyclical, which affirms that "A true ecological approach *always* becomes a social approach; it must integrate questions of justice in debates on the environment, so as to hear *both the cry of the earth and the cry of the poor*"

(Pope Francis 2015, p.49). President Obama backed him in a 2015 speech to the United Nations:

> All of our countries will be affected by a changing climate. But the world's poorest people will bear the heaviest burden—from rising seas and more intense droughts, shortages of water and food. We will be seeing climate change refugees. As His Holiness Pope Francis has rightly implored the world, this is a moral calling. (Hale 2015, p.1)

Issues of conscience require us to take a personal values inventory. Social rights activist Desmond Tutu reminds us, "If you are neutral in situations of injustice, you have chosen the side of the oppressor" (Powell and Smith 2011, p.3). While climate change issues are massive and complex, we can always continue to explore whether we are doing our part. Are we living in alignment with the values we claim? This kind of exploration often raises the theme of forgiveness as part of building integrity, and the worksheet at the end of the chapter provides several forgiveness practices that include self-compassion.

Climate-induced anxiety and depression

As we commonly see in clinical practice, depression and anxiety are cousins: they frequently co-exist and share overlapping symptoms. Many of the selective serotonin reuptake inhibitors (SSRIs) are effective in treating anxiety and depression by activating several of the same neurotransmitters (Nutt 2004). Anxiety can result from prolonged depression and vice versa. For these reasons, the clinical themes discussed here will be grouped to address both of these symptom constellations.

In Chapter 2, we explored climate-change-induced grief, but when does grief morph into depression? Helplessness, hopelessness, and isolation have long been identified as key factors in depression, and the sheer magnitude of climate change issues can easily trigger these reactions. Watch for whether your clients are isolating, shunning support, or feeling disconnected from others. When the climate grief experience fails to resolve, and there is a prolonged disruption to the client's daily life, it may be an indicator of depression.

Anxiety tends to be future-oriented, arising out of our mental "What if…?" scenarios. With much of the climate change news projecting what dire events may occur in the coming decades, we are all living with an ongoing threat of climate-change-related disruptions. This news creates ambient stress that readily fuels anxiety. The anxiety can be reinforced as we experience small changes: an earlier start to summer, driving past rivers gone dry, seeing trees dying at our favorite camping spot (Bell *et al.* 2001). If we really take in the subtle environmental changes, we can be powerfully affected—but because in some areas it is not yet strongly impacting the local population, it can also be easy to ignore.

As we have seen with climate denial, we tend to tune out non-acute signs. We become dismissive toward warnings, treating them like low-level background noise, or we quickly attribute the changes to reasons other than global warming. Denial is an unconscious survival mechanism, so we let the signs go unnoticed to avoid feeling the anxiety, and we begin to habituate to them (Bechtel and Churchman 2002). This is a very dangerous trend, and it is essential to our wellbeing—and perhaps our very survival—to understand the distinction between habituating and adapting.

When we habituate to something unhealthy, it perpetuates and worsens the problem. When change is gradual, as climate change is in some regions, we often miss "decision-trigger" opportunities that we would immediately notice with more abrupt disturbances. To understand unhealthy habituation, consider how we might sit in the sun for hours, enjoying the soothing warmth, and completely ignoring that eventually we will get sunburned. Over the course of the day we are habituating to the pleasant sensations and overlooking the facts. This is a very different reaction from the immediate, decisive action we take when an open flame moves close to our skin.

Adaptation, in contrast, means *consciously* responding to change, whether it is subtle or dramatic, using our discernment to choose the best direction after considering multiple factors. It requires being awake, being willing to have our eyes and hearts wide open, and being willing to make choices from a place of mindful awareness. It also requires flexibility to adjust and correct our course as change continues.

A key challenge with mental health issues and climate change is that many of the triggers—for example, increased heat, severe storms, and more polluted air—occur in prolonged or repetitive cycles. We cannot expect the stressors to recede into the past because we will be required to adapt to new landscapes and lifestyles.

Psychological resiliency

Resiliency is our capacity to face and handle life's challenges with flexibility and creativity, and it relies on a set of skills and perceptions that can be cultivated with practice. Resilient people share three characteristics: "A belief that they can influence life events; a tendency to find meaningful purpose in life's turmoil; and a conviction that they can learn from both positive and negative experiences" (Ripley 2009, p.91). The good news is that these qualities can be developed, and with what we are learning about the neuroplasticity of the brain, with practice we can rewire our responses so that we will consistently respond with a greater sense of clarity and calm (Graham 2013).

While there are many resiliency practices throughout this book, one of the best requires putting the book down and stepping outside. Ecopsychology places therapeutic theory and practice in an ecological context. It upholds the notion that "nature heals" as one of the oldest and most useful therapeutic tenets. Research is now tracking changes in brain physiology that confirm that we are physically and mentally more healthy when we interact regularly with nature.

People who live in urban areas have higher rates of depression than those in more rural environments. Those with access to nearby natural settings have been found to be healthier overall (Gardner 2009). But it is not just fresh air, the exercise benefits of a walk, or upping your natural dose of solar vitamin D that matters. There is something more subtle, powerful, and compelling that occurs as we are increasingly alienated from nature.

Ancient wisdom

For millennia, many indigenous traditions have been describing the emotional sustenance we derive from nature. The Nuu-chah-nulth, the First Nations peoples living on the west coast of Vancouver Island, Canada, speak of the "Hishuk Tsawalk," translated as "Everything is one, everything is connected" (Happynook 2005, p.1). Within this community it is understood that cultural diversity and biodiversity cannot be separated: they co-exist on the same continuum physically, emotionally, and spiritually.

Indigenous traditions understand health as a dynamic state that requires harmonious relationships between body, mind, spirit/soul, *and* environment. Historically, many Native American personal health assessments have included inquiries into the patient's environmental health: "Are the salmon in your rivers ill?" (Cohen 2006, p.308). Traditional healing restores balance between the person, community, and nature. And yet Ahmed Djoghlaf, the former United Nations Executive Secretary on The Convention for Biological Diversity, cited a European survey that found that 60 percent of the population did not even know the meaning of the word "biodiversity" (Zeller 2010), much less understand its importance.

Modern findings

Because more and more research is validating a link between the natural environment and our mental health, it should come as no surprise that as alienation from nature increases, so does depression. With more than half of the world's population living in cities, many people go through the day with little to no contact with the natural world. The Environmental Protection Agency (EPA) reported that 93 percent of our lives take place inside buildings or vehicles, and "Many children now spend less than 30 minutes *per week* playing outside" (Campbell 2016, p.1). Sadly, by the time children attend kindergarten, most have watched more than 5,000 hours of television—more time than it takes to earn a college degree (McDonough 2009)!

Our understanding of the mental health benefits of being in nature is multifaceted and evolving. The *Journal of Environmental Psychology* published a study suggesting that natural settings activate the parasympathetic nervous system associated with the relaxation response and the replenishment of physical and emotional energy (Ulrich *et al.* 1991). Another report, from Deakin University (Maller *et al.* 2005), found that an experience of nature increases activity in the right hemisphere of the brain. Because our urban activities are strongly analytical or left-hemisphere-dominant, nature is vital to restoring balance to the function of the brain as a whole.

Poetically, we could say that being in nature wakes up our ancestral roots, those instincts tuned to the earth rhythms of the seasons. Some part of us recognizes that our planet's ecosystem is the essential currency on which all life depends. Perhaps when we see the roots of trees growing into a stream and the leaves tipping upward to be nurtured by the sun, it is easy to recognize the way that life self-organizes into a functional, interdependent whole. In the words of Joseph Campbell, "The goal of life is to make your heartbeat match the beat of the universe, to match your nature with Nature" (Campbell and Osbon 1995, p.148). I think that some part of us, down in our bones, simply recognizes nature as "home."

The instructions for a restorative nature meditation are simple: go outside and be present. While these guidelines may sound obvious, it is not always easy if we are out of practice. It is an active mindfulness practice.

EYE-OPEN NATURE MEDITATION— COME TO YOUR SENSES

- **Listen** to the sounds: the breeze, water, birds. What sounds are nearest to you, and what is the farthest thing you can hear?

- **Smell** any scents carried in the air: soil, flowers, water.

- **Feel** the air on your skin. Is it cool or warm? Notice how it feels to breathe in the freshness. What about the texture of the grass, sand, or tree bark...feel whatever you are directly in contact with.

- **See** the colors in the sky, plants, earth. How many shades of green, yellow, blue, and brown can you distinguish?

- **Welcome** the felt-sense of the qualities you are experiencing while connected to nature, allowing them to imprint themselves in your body, mind, and emotions.

Trio of psychological climate distress themes

There are three additional clinical issues to watch for that frequently accompany psychological distress prompted by climate change: vicarious traumatization, survivor guilt, and recovery fatigue.

VICARIOUS TRAUMATIZATION

Vicarious trauma (VT) (Pearlman and Saakvitne 1995) is the cumulative emotional impact that results from empathetic engagement with traumatic experiences. It is also known as compassion fatigue and secondary traumatic stress (Stamm 1997). While most of the studies on VT have focused on therapists, volunteers, and first responders working in crisis environments, it is now applicable to the wider population as more and more people witness the climate-change-induced trauma of loved ones, communities, species, and lands. As we are exposed to more stories of loss and suffering, our own experience of pain, fear, and terror can be triggered that mirror what trauma survivors have endured. This reaction is enhanced with clients who have their own trauma history.

Symptoms of VT are extensive, and can include feeling emotionally exhausted, over or under eating, insomnia, and lingering feelings of anger and sadness at the plight of the victims. There can be an over identification with the client, with rescue fantasies or intrusive imagery of the horror, sometimes manifesting with somatic symptoms, such as stomach or head pain. This tense preoccupation can impact trust and intimacy, and interfere with maintaining life responsibilities (Pearlman and Saakvitne 1995; Rothschild 2006).

Clinical treatment includes normalizing the experience and encouraging clients to be gentle with themselves, followed by a gradual individuation that separates them from the merged identification. You can provide support by helping them to set limits on the time they spend on traumatic news, while increasing self-care practices like breath work, exercise, time in nature, and mindfulness to reduce rumination. Individual and social activities that are life-enhancing can be gradually increased until a balance is achieved. It can be helpful to offer education about the distinction between empathy and compassion outlined in Chapter 2.

SURVIVOR GUILT

Survivor guilt, also known as survivor syndrome, can be experienced from afar as well as by those directly touched by climate change loss: "Why them (or their home, etc.) and not me/mine? Could I have done more? I do not deserve to be spared." There can also be guilt about what an individual did to save themselves in a crisis—such as follow their instinct to flee, but then later ponder whether they should have stayed to help others. Guilt can also be triggered if they were unsuccessful in their attempts to save a person, pet, or property. Survival guilt may be an unconscious way to try to build a sense of belonging to the culture or group that experienced the event and an attempt to provide justice and security in the face of unanswerable questions and mind-numbing catastrophes (Danieli 1984; Klein 1968).

Using the therapeutic approaches consistent with your training, it can be useful to examine whether our client's survival guilt is reactivating early childhood beliefs of unworthiness. Processing often irrational beliefs can have some benefit if the client has not explored their thoughts, and they can gain strength over time by living with the unanswerable, existential "why" questions. Satisfaction often comes from assisting the client to create meaning from an adverse event. They can choose what it means to live their life with purpose, making the best of what their life can be. Many people reassess what is valuable to them, and find that becoming engaged with climate causes can be a tribute to those who suffered loss and reduce the chances of it happening again to others.

Recovery fatigue

We have seen that when climate change disaster strikes, the initial focus is on basic needs including safety and access to food, shelter, and medical needs, as well as addressing the accompanying emotional distress. It does not take long for physical and mental exhaustion to develop: adjusting to everything being new and different, processing one's losses, and the sheer overexertion from working toward restoration. Recovery fatigue includes all the thoughts and feelings that accompany the sentiment, "When is this going to be over?!"

Even with the beauty and resiliency that can emerge from the heart of devastating events, there is tremendous ongoing struggle during recovery, and the timeline can be prolonged depending on the degree of impact to the area and the available resources. If we take a look at a thin slice of the recovery timeline from Hurricane Katrina, we can get a glimpse of just how exhausting the long-term needs really are.

The amount of federal aid provided to Louisiana was not proportional to the degree of damage, and two years post-Katrina New Orleans had only 58 percent of its population back (*The Economist* 2007). Cleanup efforts resulted in elevated levels of lead, arsenic, and other toxic chemicals spread throughout the urban area. At the five-year recovery point, there were significantly higher mold spore counts in flooded areas, and 80 percent of the local children with asthma were sensitive to mold, three times the national average (Mulvihill 2010). Ten years post-Katrina some people were still living in FEMA-provided trailers and mobile homes (Smith 2015a). Recovery fatigue can compromise our ability to use our best judgment, and we often react more slowly or demonstrate confusion. Fatigue also diminishes our ability to concentrate, which reduces motivation and makes us more forgetful (Sonnentag and Zijlstra 2006; Betancourt *et al.* 2009).

Just as the recovery of infrastructure is long-term, so is the psychological healing. Treatment approaches that strengthen both internal and external coping strategies provide the best results. Internal approaches include normalizing, increasing mindfulness, and resiliency-building practices. External support involves providing information about additional aid programs and boosting family and social resources to strengthen the client's outer structure.

Coping with an increase in illnesses

Because we are part of nature, good health requires a thriving biosphere. The University College London-Lancet Commission describes climate change as, "The biggest global health threat of the 21st century," (Costello *et al.* 2009, p.1), and it predicts that the health and wellbeing of billions of people will be at risk (Costello *et al.* 2009). Health-related consequences result from five aspects of climate-induced environmental change: temperature extremes, poor air quality, vector-borne diseases, water-related illnesses, and food safety and distribution (Balbus *et al.* 2016).

TEMPERATURE EXTREMES

Climate scientists project that extreme heat events in the United States will become more frequent and longer lasting. Severe heat waves that used to occur every 20 years could happen as often as every two to four years (Karl, Melillo, and Peterson 2009). In 2003, a heat wave in Europe led to 70,000 deaths in a single summer (Robine *et al.* 2008). Between 2004 and 2013, there was a 61 percent increase in the number of deaths in India due to heat stroke, although there are indications that the incidence is vastly underreported (Mallapur 2015). In addition to the more obvious heat-related health impacts, temperature extremes can also exacerbate chronic conditions including cardiovascular disease, respiratory disease, cerebrovascular disease, and diabetes-related conditions (Balbus *et al.* 2016).

AIR QUALITY

Chronic respiratory diseases are the third leading cause of death in the United States, and breathing-related conditions are expected to become one of the most fast-growing health problems over the coming decades. From 1980 to 2010, deaths from chronic lung diseases have already increased by 50 percent as global air pollution continues to worsen. According to a 2016 report by the World Health Organization (WHO) that covers 3,000 cities in 103 countries, more than 80 percent of people living in urban areas that monitor air pollution are exposed to air quality levels that exceed the recommended limits (WHO 2016). In addition, warmer temperatures are creating record-high pollen counts that have increased the incidence of asthma attacks and intensified allergic sensitivity (Bernstein and Rice 2013).

VECTOR-BORNE DISEASES

Vector-borne diseases transmitted by mosquitoes, ticks, and fleas are sensitive to temperature fluctuations. We have a recent example in the changing ecosystems that support the spread of the Zika virus. The species of mosquito that transmits Zika can also spread West Nile virus, dengue, and chickungunya. Kathryn Jacobsen, Professor of Global Health at George Mason University, states:

> Changes in temperature, precipitation, and humidity can alter how long the mosquitoes live, how often they bite, how many offspring they have, and how quickly a virus reproduces inside an infected mosquito, and each of those changes can mean more humans are exposed to mosquitoes. (Mercer 2016, p.1)

WATER-RELATED ILLNESSES

Water is at risk as well, with an increase in water-related contaminants that cause illness. It is anticipated that there will be a growing need for beach closures with restrictions on harvesting shellfish. In 2015, crab season was banned in the states of California, Oregon, and Washington due to a toxic algae bloom created from warmer ocean temperatures (Mitchell 2015). Parts of the ocean are losing oxygen, which will likely be widespread by 2030 or 2040. These significant impacts on marine ecosystems will leave some areas of ocean uninhabitable for certain species (D'Angelo 2016).

Unless you live in an affected area, you may not be aware that there have been many "boil drinking water" orders in effect in 2016 in multiple United States states; a few include parts of New Hampshire (New Hampshire Department of Environmental Services 2016), West Virginia (West Virginia American Water 2016), Ohio (Ohio Environmental Protection Agency 2016), Washington (Washington State Department of Health 2016), California (Bienick 2016), Massachusetts (Massachusetts Department of Environmental Protection 2016), New York (Clinton County Health Department 2016), Georgia (Key 2016), and Texas (Fort Worth Water Department 2016). While incidents of water contamination are not new, climate change increases the complexity of keeping drinking water safe. That is because there are numerous factors involved, including flooding, fracking, and contamination due to water-pressure shifts when reservoirs hit record-low levels.

FOOD SAFETY AND AVAILABILITY

A report released in December of 2015 entitled *Climate Change, Global Food Security, and U.S. Food System* was written by a consortium of authors from 19 federal, academic, nongovernmental, and intergovernmental organizations in four countries whose goal was to identify the likely effects of climate change on global food security through 2100. One of the report's conclusions is that "Climate change is very likely to affect global, regional, and local food security by disrupting food availability, decreasing access to food, and making utilization more difficult" (Brown *et al.* 2015, p.ix). Not only will extreme temperatures and water distribution have the obvious impacts on food production, there will also be secondary issues such as increased plant diseases and pests and degradation of soil quality, which influence the nutritional benefits of our food.

GUIDED IMAGERY: MIND–BODY SKILLS TO SUPPORT HEALTH AND WELLBEING

While our primary efforts are to halt and reverse climate change, we must also address the growing needs that the environmental crisis is creating and study effective adaptation models. To address the mental health problems that are accompanying the increase in climate-change-induced health issues, guided imagery is effective for cultivating both physiological and emotional resiliency. Martin Rossman, M.D., a physician and leading expert in medical guided imagery, summarizes its value:

> [Guided imagery] has been shown to be helpful in medical conditions as diverse as acute and chronic pain, sleep disorders, allergies, asthma, fertility and childbirth, anxiety, depression, stress management, cancer treatment, medical decision-making, preparing for and recovering from medical and surgical procedures, and more. Imagery can be a potent way to influence patient attitudes, expectations, motivation for change, and ability to cope with difficult medical events. It can be a helpful diagnostic aid and a tool for engaging and empowering patients in their own care. (Davenport 2016, p.84)

Although it requires training in guided imagery in order to apply some of the more complex imagery processes to clients' medical conditions, this foundational mind–body tool called "Peaceful Place" is a useful practice to provide respite from medically induced stress and calm the nervous system. It serves the dual purpose of supporting the body's natural ability to heal and providing emotional relief.

All forms of guided imagery require an internal state of "active receptivity." Beginning each exercise with a relaxation process allows our most habitual thought patterns to loosen, making room for images and impressions to arise from the deeper levels that lie beneath our conscious awareness. The images are often surprising to the client, yet they "make sense." For example, after I describe the Peaceful Place exercise, it's common for clients to reply, "Oh great, I'll go to my favorite beach on Kauai," or "I've done this before, my peaceful place is a cabin in the woods." While those settings may in fact appear during the exercise, often that person will report something like this: "I haven't been here in more than 20 years, but I'm finding myself on my grandmother's farm. It's so comforting to be sitting on her porch and smelling her cooking coming from the kitchen. I'm amazed, but it feels wonderful."

The reason that unexpected images can emerge is that prior to the exercise, the person's thinking mind was busy making a plan based on past experience and choosing something already known to be associated with a pleasant feeling. Maybe there's a sense of freedom at the beach or protection at the cabin. In this example, the image shifted when a deeper part of the person recognized that the feeling of *comfort* associated with the farm was a better match for the experience they truly desired in that moment. Sometimes the peaceful place a client imagines is completely unknown to them: a lush waterfall in a cove they have never visited brings on a specific felt-sense that perfectly fulfills a present need. Using words like, *"Allow (or invite)* an image to form" supports a state of receptive awareness—rather than, *"Find (or pick)* a place that you find relaxing," which specifically asks for experiences from the client's conscious mind.

SAFETY PRECAUTIONS

Peaceful Place is a mind–body imagery practice that can lower blood pressure, which is a benefit for many clients. However, some medical conditions or medications create low or unstable blood pressure, in which case this practice would be contraindicated without skilled modifications being made to the practice, which would come with imagery training. And while guided imagery is very effective with resolving trauma, there are very specific protocols for that clinical application. If a client has unresolved trauma, this practice could loosen their familiar defenses and prompt emotional flooding.

If the peaceful place the client imagines is an environment that has suffered a climate catastrophe, acknowledge their distress and then ask the client to invite in a different, uncompromised setting for the practice. Assure them that you can work together on their experience of loss whenever they like, but for now find out if they are able to engage in this resiliency practice. It can be very helpful to the grief and trauma process to explore loss using imagery, but that is a complex clinical intervention that serves a different purpose than the Peaceful Place exercise.

The practice would also be contraindicated for clients with psychotic tendencies or who experience severe dissociation. In your assessment, you will need to make a clinical determination whether this is an appropriate practice given these guidelines.[1]

Peaceful Place

Begin by briefly describing to the client what this relaxation practice involves and acquire their consent to give it a try before proceeding. Answer any questions they have, and let them know that they can speak aloud to you or even open their eyes at any time. Assure them that there is no "right way" to do the exercise—it is just a way to explore relaxation.

Read each section at a relaxed pace, taking time to pause and allow the client to deepen their experience and engage with the images that arise. Start with reading "Progressive Relaxation" found in the Appendix, and then continue with the script below.

Now invite an image to form of a place or an environment that can support your relaxation or even deepen it. This peaceful and safe place could be indoors or outdoors, familiar to you or imaginary, as long as it is comfortable, beautiful, and inviting to you. Once it begins to take shape, notice the colors you are most aware of and textures. What time of day does it seem to be? I wonder if you can tell what season it is? What are the aromas or scents in the air, or perhaps there is just a freshness? Notice any sounds that are part of this place, or if it has a particular quality of silence. Take some time to explore this beautiful place, and then pick a spot where you would like to enjoy this safe and peaceful place the most, whether standing, sitting, reclining, or continuing to explore. If there is anything at all that you want or need that would help you feel even more comfortable, make those adjustments now.

Notice how you feel being in your peaceful place and the particular qualities you experience. Let yourself be nourished by the beauty and ease. Allow any qualities that feel good or beneficial to become part of your breathing, so that as you inhale, you bring the peaceful feeling of this place and any other enjoyable qualities into your body. Let the peacefulness ride along with the oxygen that travels to every cell in your body, head to toe. Infuse your body with the beauty of this place, so that it is all around you and within you. You are not only here, you are a part of this beautiful environment.

Imagine letting the peacefulness fill your mind and your heart—allow the best qualities to infuse every layer of who you are.

We will take a few moments in silence to simply enjoy being here. Feel completely free to use this time in your beautiful place in whatever way appeals to you, as long as it is comfortable and relaxing (pause for about one minute). If this place has a message for you, something it wants you to know, what would it be?

As we prepare to bring this practice to a close, know that you can return here in a similar way at any time. Know also that—just like a delicious meal whose nutrition continues to help you after the meal is over—the beneficial relaxation from this time also continues with you. Feel any valuable shifts that have occurred, whether your body feels more relaxed, or your mind or emotions more peaceful. Remain aware of these beneficial changes while you also sense the room around you, noticing as the sounds register in the room. Feel the movement of your breath, and stretch out into your hands, feet, and to the top of your head. Remain connected to the peacefulness while you begin to notice the light in the room through your closed eyelids, and the temperature of the air on your skin. When you feel ready, taking the time you need, stay connected with the peacefulness and open your eyes.

Ask the client how they feel, and invite them to share anything they would like to about their experience. Encourage them to practice Peaceful Place imagery on their own, or get support by listening to a recording that would guide them in a similar way. It can also be helpful to draw or write about their experience to integrate it even more fully.

Faced with climate disruptions large and small, we can reach into the depths of ourselves to cultivate resiliency and embody our evolving role with humanity and our living earth. As Helen Keller so aptly stated, "Although the world is full of suffering, it is also full of overcoming it" (Keller 1933, p.6). We can learn to see again, with our hearts, who we are capable of being. We can deepen the connections with ourselves, cultivate relational intelligence with each other, and protect the home we love. We can open ourselves and our clients to perceive in new ways, aligning our skills, gifts, and lifestyles in an ecoharmonious way.

Additional resources

Buzzell, L. and Chalquist, C. (eds) (2009) *Ecotherapy: Healing with Nature in Mind.* San Francisco, CA: Sierra Club Books.

Chalquist, C. (2007) *Terrapsychology: Reengaging the Soul of Place.* New Orleans, LA: Spring Journal Books.

Eisenstein, C. (2013) *The More Beautiful World Our Hearts Know is Possible.* Berkeley, CA: North Atlantic Books.

Weller, F. (2015) *The Wild Edge of Sorrow.* Berkeley, CA: North Atlantic Books.

WORKSHEET
Moral injury—forgiving ourselves, forgiving others

It is easy to confuse forgiveness of both oneself and others with:

- condoning a damaging action

- minimizing valid feelings

- fear that your story will be lost

- not standing up for justice

- dismissing the need for accountability.

There may even be some wrongs so heinous that they fall outside our conventional framework for repairing moral relations, and no one other than you can decide whether forgiveness is warranted.

Consider too that it serves no one, and corrects no injustice, to be in a self-constructed prison of rage, self-deprecation, resentment, or shame. Paul Boese, a World War II veteran, wisely said, "Forgiveness does not change the past, but it does enlarge the future" (Kassinove and Tafrate 2002, p.244.) Forgiveness paves the way for ethical action that can support self-growth and contribute to making the world a better place. Forgiveness is layered and takes time, but these practices can be beneficial steps within a longer process. It is recommended that non-professionals reading this book work with their mental health practitioner to explore the feelings and options that arise from exploring this worksheet.

Forgiving oneself

Making amends with others is an excellent step toward self-forgiveness. It is more than offering an apology—it includes taking action to restore, directly if possible, something that we damaged. For example, if we ridiculed someone in the past for their environmental protection efforts, which we thought of as "fanaticism," but now we realize the significance of their work, we can do more than just apologize; if possible, we also join them, or become involved in similar green efforts.

1. Identify an incident that you want to repair.

2. Brainstorm ways to amend it, and write the steps and timeline for following through.

_____

_____

_____

_____

_____

_____

_____

Forgiving others

There is a natural emotional process that may traverse the full spectrum of feelings when we have been harmed—but we sometimes dig a neurological groove that traps us in an emotional loop. It can feel safe to justify being right, and anger emphasizes our point. We may mistake rage for outrage. Sometimes we get stuck because we have not yet honored some aspect of ourselves, such as attending to the hurt hidden under the anger. The truth is that we are practicing forgiveness for our own healing.

What if we viewed our offenders as being lost in delusion? What if their wrongdoing came from a history of their own suffering that hardened into a belief system? Or what if we bear the mystery of the unanswerable "Why?" In experimenting with these ways of seeing, we are not excusing the person's culpability, but the process does increase our own compassion. It summons our courage to face life's losses and step into our own loving nature. Forgiveness is a powerful and crucial process for enhancing the wellbeing of not only ourselves, but also the children of today and tomorrow.

Feel free to modify the script below to match what you are ready to experience. The opening paragraph of the Forgiveness Meditation can be replaced with the Peaceful Place script for a more in-depth meditation.

Forgiveness Meditation[2]

Sit comfortably, close your eyes, and bring your awareness to the center of your chest. Breathe with ease for about three minutes, as though your breath could move directly in and out of your heart, as you allow your mind and body to relax. Feel yourself present in this moment, right now.

Breathing gently into the area of your heart, let yourself feel all the gripping, weight, and hardened barriers that have formed from the pain you have experienced. Look upon your own heart with tenderness and kind regard for how much pain you have been carrying.

Acknowledge the ways that continuing to carry this pain is like allowing an arrow to remain in your heart, instead of removing it. Realize that it is you who is suffering, and that releasing the pain, grudges, and resentments is a gift to yourself.

Knowing that you are safe, here and now, let yourself feel what your heart is holding. Invite emotions to flow to the surface and be released.

If you feel ready, if you feel a "yes" inside your heart, call to mind the people who have harmed you that you want to forgive. Tell them how much they hurt you and why you feel the way you do. Take the time you need.

If it feels true to you right now, affirm that you have carried this pain long enough, and say, "I offer you forgiveness. To the best of my ability, I will not knowingly allow this to happen again. I am ready and willing to allow past hurts to heal."

Now allow the image of those people to dissolve and bring your focus back to your own heart. Continue to breathe tenderly into your heart, and notice any shifts or changes.

Let your soothing breath now radiate from your heart out into your entire body, filling it from head to toe with a sense of ease, freedom, and comfort. Continue breathing this way for a few moments.

Staying aware of anything that feels valuable or useful to you, begin to sense the room around you, and when you feel ready, open your eyes.

It is helpful to take a few moments to write or draw your experience.

Chapter 6

Resiliency Stories

It is nearly impossible to understand fully terrain we have not walked. When we hear about massive losses, we can empathize with the pain because almost all of us have experienced some kind of grief. But the resiliency, the glimmering of gold through the ashes, the tensile strength forged by extreme hardship; these may be harder to imagine if we have not lived through a climate event of significant magnitude. While not all locations have the external resources—nor all individuals the internal ones—to rebound easily, resiliency stories are common in areas impacted by climate chaos. The very frequency of resiliency themes points to the compelling strength and beauty of the human spirit. While the goal is clearly to stop and reverse the destructive consequences of climate change, these stories of hope remind us of how attainable transformative personal change can be.

Resiliency is more than just mustering the fortitude to get yourself out of bed in the morning after life has knocked down your dreams, hopes, and perhaps your house. It is reaching for something inside that's never been touched, or has gone dormant while we manage the pressing routines of our daily lives. Maybe it is rising in the morning and remembering that we are part of the world, formed of the same atoms as the soil and the stars...that the universe is all that has ever been, and our life and breath are part of it. As we watch the news, we may suddenly realize that life is both tragic and beautiful, and that we will choose beauty.

While the first story is not about a climate-change-related disaster, I found it to be a perfect illustration of one woman's resilient journey that began with multiple losses by fire. Fire is—and will become—a familiar aspect of climate change, and stories like Lori's are unfortunately projected to become more and more common. Because of the warming climate and increased drought, the number and intensity of wildfires are projected to double by late this century across 11 western states (National Wildlife Federation 2008). Hearing Lori's experience through the eyes of a 13-year-old, and then reading her reflections 30 years later, offers us a long-term view of resiliency that is unusual: most of the recognized climate-related disasters have been fairly recent.

This chapter tells resiliency stories from the viewpoints of an individual and a rural town, and it describes a host of proactive measures that test a new model of civil society and may help prevent more climate destruction. Before, during, and after climate change is addressed, let us nourish and even celebrate our inherent resiliency.

Lori Cheek

Lori's father woke in the middle of the night to an eerie silence. All year round, day and night, the Cheek household could hear the familiar hum of an old fan they used as a sound barrier to create a little extra privacy between rooms. The silence signaled that something was not right. Lori's dad assumed that there was a power outage, or that the fan had finally worn itself out, so he got up to troubleshoot—and then he saw the flames. "Wake up! Get up! Outside! NOW!" It all happened so quickly; Lori, her Mom, and her brother slipped on the nearest shoes, scrambled to grab whatever they could, and ran out the front door.

It was the coldest night that Taylorsville, Kentucky had experienced since the 1800s.

Lori, then 13 years old, clutched a doll and a photo album as she stood in the snow in pajamas and sockless shoes, trying to make sense of what was happening. "Samantha!" she cried, "We have to get Samantha!" Her loyal canine companion normally lived in the backyard, but because of the bitter cold this was one of the rare nights she was allowed to sleep in the basement. The flames and smoke made it too dangerous to go inside to retrieve her, though Lori felt willing to do almost anything to save her beloved dog. Samantha did not come out when she was called again and again.

Taylorsville is a small rural town, and it was the local volunteer fire department that responded to the call for help. They quickly set up their hoses but found them useless: the nearby water source was frozen solid. A second truck was called to try to figure out what to do. The first responders and family were stunned, helplessly watching the house become engulfed in flames. Lori's parents had collected antique furniture, and all the things they had worked for, treasured, and taken care of as a part of their home were burning in front of their eyes.

The second fire truck arrived, but it collided with the first truck on the slippery driveway. Lori and her brother pushed two family cars out of the way to prevent them from being hit or catching fire. She found a source of physical strength that, to this day, she cannot explain. At one point in the chaos it was unclear where her mother was, and when the house imploded in flames Lori thought her Mom might still be inside. Fortunately, she was okay; she was watching from one of the fire trucks. Later that night, after their home burned to its foundation, Lori and her family slept on the floor of her uncle's house.

They later learned that the fire started in the aluminum wiring in the attic and quickly spread to the roof. It jumped to the woodpile at the side of the house, perfect tinder for the merciless bonfire. The whole family was treated for smoke inhalation and frostbite. Very little was salvaged from the ashes: some of Lori's Mom's gold jewelry and a few of her brother's baseball cards, tightly bound in a tin. As terrible as it was, Lori was glad they found Samantha's remains. She explained that this helped her to grieve, and they buried the dog with a family ceremony in the backyard.

Lori described this pivotal life event to me 30 years later; the images of that night were still powerful and vivid, and she lives with the results of the frostbite she suffered on a daily basis. "Others can only feel the awful part: they can't really understand. I learned so much about life that I treasure. It shaped the values of generosity and gratitude that I live by" (Cheek, personal communication, April 18, 2016).

"I was a bratty 13-year-old at the time, but this event changed me. We lost everything we owned, but we had each other. It brought our family closer. This near-death experience made us a tight little tribe" (Cheek, personal communication, April 18, 2016). Lori also described the tremendous generosity she witnessed in her community. "A neighbor came at our request and bulldozed our entire ruins. We gave him a check and he ripped it up. The town had a shower for us filled with gifts you wouldn't even begin to imagine, from clothing, china, and silver to household electronics: pretty much everything to get us back on our feet. One of my dad's colleagues had a condo that was empty while his parents were in Florida for the winter, and we moved there with everything provided for three months, while gifts from the community kept flowing in non-stop. Our tiny town replaced as much as they could of what we'd lost. It was amazing to see the never-ending gifts everyone brought to us. We were truly blessed" (Cheek, personal communication, April 18, 2016).

They decided to rebuild on the same site, and Lori was fascinated watching the architect bring their new house back to life. It was magic made real to that 13-year-old: her family's life was being reconstructed one brick at a time, and the process was both beautiful and practical. Witnessing this act of creativity in such a personal way inspired Lori to go to architecture school, and she had a 15-year career in architecture and design.

"I live in New York now, but material possessions don't mean much to me. I don't have a room full of my childhood toys at my parent's house, but I still have that one doll that I bring out whenever I visit them and the photos. It's enough." The many values forged from that time in her life spill out: "I learned how generous and beautiful people can be, and how much relationships matter. My current job is related to building relationships. Because of the frostbite, I can't feel my toes when the temperature drops, but I'm grateful I have toes. I know that stuff is just stuff: it's life that is precious. That experience taught me that every day is a gift" (Cheek, personal communication, April 18, 2016).

Jamestown, Colorado

On September 9, 2013, a slow-moving cold front stalled over Colorado's Front Range mountains. Within three days of a non-stop deluge, flood waters had spread across an area of almost 200 miles, covering 23 counties (Aguilar 2015). The National Weather Service called it a thousand-year event (NOAA 2013)—the kind of declaration that we are now hearing on a regular basis about superstorms resulting from climate change. President Obama called a state of emergency.

Jamestown is a small community of 270 people nestled in the mountains 12 miles northwest of Boulder, and it has seen more than its share of disaster. In 2003, high winds snapped a 20-foot-tall tree that took down a 31,200-volt power line, sparking a fire that burned 3,500 acres and destroyed 12 homes in a single day (Graham *et al.* 2012). Jamestown rebuilt itself, but was hit even harder ten years later by the flood. Since the fire had destroyed many of the trees in one-third of the Fourmile Canyon Creek drainage basin, it was more susceptible to rapid runoff, contributing to the later storm and flood damage (Kroh 2013). This is an example of how climate change events are interconnected, as when drought contributes to runaway fires and warming oceans lead to toxic algae blooms that impact fisheries.

During the three-day storm, half of the town's roads were washed away and all of the underground infrastructure at Jamestown's drinking-water treatment plant was destroyed, along with 50 percent of the water distribution lines. The Jamestown Fire Station was damaged and the Town Square Park and 13 homes were transformed into debris scattered down 25 miles of riverbed. In tiny Jamestown alone, the public infrastructure loss was estimated at $20 million (Town of Jamestown 2013).

The National Guard Chinook helicopters were the only way to access the community quickly and safely, and they swooped down to the muddy lake that just days before was the town of Jamestown to evacuate 90 percent of the residents. In spite of working diligently toward recovery, three years later the impact still resounds: not all the homes have been rebuilt, and the roads are not anticipated to be fully restored before 2017.

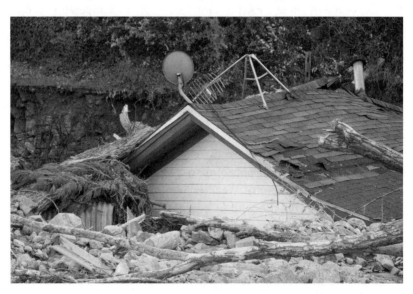

JAMESTOWN, COLORADO FLOOD 2013
PHOTO: SAL DEVINCENZO

In small towns there is a natural resiliency that is built by a shared sense of practical interdependence. During a typical winter in Jamestown, the roads are plowed by three local volunteers, with another community member contributing money for gas. This home-grown team enables everyone to have access to shops and work. The residents are interconnected, knowing that they cannot get by without each other. Their close-knit structure also creates strong collective empathy, and those who still had homes after the storm felt the stress of those who were still struggling or displaced.

As the water receded and roads were reconstructed, some residents were able to return. When the water plant was once again functional (nearly one year later), this cohesive and self-sufficient community expressed its desire to be full participants in the decision-making involved in the rebuilding efforts. Right after the flood, town hall meetings were held every two weeks with a full turnout. As the rebuilding process began in earnest, meetings about the community's losses gave way to meetings about visioning its future. It was a natural time of reevaluation: what did they want to restore to pre-flood conditions, and what could be created differently as they rebuilt? What might the future look like beyond recovery?

The residents take pride in their unique community's character, and many of them regard themselves as stewards of the natural environment. How could they design infrastructure with stronger, more resilient systems that will be financially and technologically sustainable and also have a minimal impact on the environment? These considerations were made all the more difficult because deep grief, trauma, and emotional healing from the devastating losses were occurring at the same time.

PEACE AND FOOD JUST DOWN THE ROAD

Calryn Aston is a Jamestown resident and senior teacher at the Shambhala Meditation Center in nearby Boulder. She approaches resilient recovery by uniting two of her passions: community and mindfulness. Calryn's home was not damaged in the flood, but it was six months before she had running water and could return home. She was active in the town-hall meetings and offered whatever she could to support the recovery efforts.

Calryn worked with the Boulder Shambhala Meditation Center to open its doors to the community as a gathering place for both inner and outer nourishment. It was a team effort, with many volunteers eager to serve. For two days, shortly after the Jamestown evacuation, the Center's community room was transformed, piled high with free groceries and empty boxes and bags for easy transport. Mike Glass, manager of a local Whole Foods Market and also a member of the Center, generously arranged for food donations (Aston 2014).

Another form of nourishment was plentiful: tables and chairs were arranged so that displaced Jamestown community members could comfortably gather and take time to be with each other. FEMA counselors were also present, continuing to access and respond to community needs.

Everyone was welcomed with kindness and warmth when they arrived at the Center. Tender conversations were supported by a beautiful, peaceful environment. In the best possible way, the atmosphere was contagious, with calm resilience seemingly transmitted by the place itself. Some people spontaneously inquired about the location of the meditation hall and asked if they could use it.

With mindfulness, how you are present with people becomes as powerful as what you might say or do, and the genuine compassion of presence opens a window to our own resilient nature. Calryn describes her experience of the two-day gathering:

> There was a lot of listening with a great sense of care and presence. There was room to express both what hurt and what could be appreciated. I find that in mindfully attending to themselves and others, people naturally recover their own insights and strength. And when a group is connected in this way, a lot can happen. (Calryn Aston, personal communication, March 31, 2016)

While this kind of devastation can push people to a soul-shaking precipice, there is palpable strength to be found in community. Deep connections make it easier to manage our difficulties, and the experience of caring calls forth deeper internal resources.

Only a week after the flood, some residents aspired to have meditation become a regular part of their community, right alongside the infrastructure planning and meeting their food and transportation needs. There are now weekly meditation meetings in Jamestown and a larger periodic Contemplative Writing gathering where experiences are shared through meditation, intentional dialogue, and writing.

Mental health voucher system

For all Boulder County residents impacted by the flood, the Foothills United Way offered a wonderful model of individualized mental health care by providing vouchers for free psychotherapy for anyone who needed it. Qualified residents were given a pre-printed voucher for the therapist of their choice to fill out and be reimbursed for services rendered, up to a defined amount. The therapists were paid their customary fee up to $200 per appointment. Residents struggling with fear, anger, insomnia, anxiety, and other symptoms found this service tremendously helpful. About 500 people in Jamestown and surrounding communities participated in the program, and efforts are being made now to re-extend the offer to those still healing from trauma (United Way 2014).

The road less traveled

Many organizations were involved in the recovery efforts, including FEMA, United Way, the American Red Cross, the Salvation Army, and the Flatirons Rotary Club. Getting to and from Jamestown continued to be a challenge, with many of the roadways either completely washed away or unsafe to drive. A temporary route ran right through the sleepy little town of Gold Hill. Many people used it to get to work or bring home staples that were no longer locally available. Aid organizations drove through to bring in equipment and supplies. Drivers from Jamestown were very conscious of how much the Gold Hill residents value their quiet, and they were aware of the new source of heavy traffic through the nearby town. They watched as the road dust began to coat store windows. Many of the Jamestown commuters felt terrible for disrupting their neighboring town, but there was no other alternative. Pam Sherman lives just outside Gold Hill and heard about the concerns. She told one local resident, "We were so glad to be able to do something useful. Everyone here would have done anything to help" (Sherman, personal communication, January 29, 2016).

Normal boundaries and priories shift during disaster recovery. Privacy breaks down when we respond to other people's needs. Strangers were let into homes to use bathrooms, something that would normally be deemed rude or even dangerous. When faced with such an extreme level of shared distress, we stop seeing each other as strangers and instead we become simply fellow human beings who share the same aspirations, fears, and needs. No one took advantage of the many ways that people offered to help each other, and generosity became the natural response.

FROM THE MOUTHS OF BABES

In 2010, Lynda Jean Bell moved to Jamestown and enrolled in a Ph.D. program at the University of Colorado to further her career in atmospheric and ocean sciences. It was not long before the town learned that Lynda is also a musician and music teacher, and the enthusiasm from the community soon inspired her to start a singing and songwriting class with a group of enthusiastic four- and five-year-old mountain kids. The class of anywhere from 8 to 14 children love to write and sing about their life in the mountains—what it is like to live among rivers, trees, and bears, and a favorite song called "Home Sweet Home" has the audience joining in when they perform at local festivals and gatherings. They proudly named themselves the "Wild Mountain Kids." The classes are a strong, joyful, kid-style way of forming skills and bonds of friendship, confidence, fun, and celebrating "home."

When the flood struck two years later, Jamestown was literally torn in two, with a chasm opening across the center of town that prevented passage and divided the community. With most of the town evacuated, the kids were also separated from each other, which generated tremendous fear and great concern for their close friends. There was a period of time when communication systems were down, and there was no way to learn of each other's location or condition.

The families who remained in the community during the flood recovery wanted to create a supportive structure for the kids there, and a local family opened their home to become a one-room schoolhouse for the upcoming year. They re-established the school schedule and curriculum, and Lynda became the school's temporary music teacher. The kids continued to write and sing about their lives, but the songs now included tears, worries, and hopes resulting from the flood. The power of music to express and heal deep emotions was already a direct and natural experience for these children. One song talks about the "little bridge that brightened the way," referring to a wooden structure temporarily constructed across the chasm. Another lyric includes these hopeful words, "The playground is still there!" Young children have a natural receptivity and resiliency that lets in all of what is occurring around them, so they also wrote songs about rainbows, blue skies, and the season's holidays.

Now together again, the kids continue to write and perform together. Bob Tarantino, music producer with Tolstar Goat House Studio, heard the kids singing at local mountain gatherings and recognized how special they are. He proposed producing a CD, and with the financial support of charities and the community Tolstar released "The Wild Mountain Kids, Here in Jamestown" in 2016. Proceeds from the sales will support the Traditional Mountain Area Children's Music Program, and will help purchase instruments to expand the music program at Jamestown Elementary School. Now everyone can hear the sounds of heart-strong resiliency and joy as the Wild Mountain Kids sing about their home: "Where blue skies will shine again, and people will sparkle once again. I still believe in it, here in Jamestown" (Bell, personal communication, May 26, 2016).

HUMOR AS A RESILIENCY SKILL

Resiliency comes in many forms, often surprising us, and laughter can help us get through difficult times. Fran Etzkorn is an elder living in Longmont, a city east of Boulder, who was eager to help with the cleanup, but a serious medical condition prevented her from doing strenuous physical labor. As people shoveled mud and carried moldy furnishings and clothes out of their waterlogged homes, Fran laced up her boots and took to the road pushing a brand-new wheelbarrow she had purchased with a purpose: it was filled with chocolates.

"Chocolate, chocolate!" she called, and her neighbors swarmed out of their homes like bees to honey. But when they came to the chocolate wheelbarrow, they discovered they could not eat: their hands were filthy. So Fran would unwrap the pieces they pointed to and feed them (Sherman, personal communication, January 29, 2016). In more ways than one, there were many sweet exchanges. The incongruous mix of muck and delicacies was so unexpected that everyone was laughing at the absurdity of the situation. Neighbors continue to retell this story, generating a laugh, a smile, and a feeling of warm connection.

Meanwhile Jamestown is still on the mend, but the physical infrastructure is already stronger than it was before the flood. Households are more resilient, and the town has upgraded its telephone, electricity, fire, and water systems. The community is even more closely bonded: those who were isolated are less so, and there are more vectors of communication available. The community members not only recognize how much they need each other, they also deeply value their collective strength and are empowered by it.

Proactive climate resiliency

There are many innovative individuals, programs, and organizations that are working to build resiliency and even reverse climate change. You will find four themes woven throughout most of the examples below: local sourcing, renewable energy, overall reduced consumption, and waste reduction.

We may not be aware of the hidden but high environmental costs to our clothes, food, and other products that are shipped from overseas from the pollution that results from their transport. In addition, social justice issues are often embedded, including the slave labor recently uncovered in the Thai shrimp market (Krystal 2015) and the extreme abuses of factory workers in Cambodia who produce labels for popular brands like Gap and Adidas (Winn 2015). Many of the movements that urge us toward local production can help us break away from our high-consumption, single-use, plastic-ridden culture that is polluting the land, sky, and seas. Did you know that the amount of plastic currently in the oceans exceeds the amount of plankton six times over? (Andrews 2012.)

The connections are so interwoven in our daily choices and lifestyles that it can be overwhelming. Long-time environmentalist and Executive Director of Project Drawdown Paul Hawken reveals the other side of the coin: we are awakening to the problems and making change on a huge scale. In his book *Blessed Unrest: How the Largest Social Movement in History is Restoring Grace, Justice, and Beauty to the World*, he estimates that there are up to two million ecologically sustainable and social justice non-profit organizations active worldwide (Hawken 2008).

Emphasizing the power of collective action builds confidence that change is possible. There are examples of individuals who were once unconvinced of the reality of climate change who are now willing to leave a positive legacy by participating in environmental actions, because they believe that mitigation efforts will have a positive overall effect on society (Van Zomeren, Spears, and Leach 2010). Any group that provides a creative and educational forum for sharing what can be done and what others are doing can help create new social norms, an important feature of inspiring others to become involved. Here are just a few examples of the countless creative solutions that are rapidly emerging around the world.

REBUILDING GREEN

In 2007, Greensburg, Kansas, was flattened by a two-mile-wide tornado that travelled for 22 miles on the ground. In the recovery effort, all of the city buildings were built to the platinum standards of the Leadership in Energy and Environmental Design certification guideline (LEED). Greensburg is the first city in the nation to undertake such an ambitious plan from the ground up, so to speak. This has made the city true to its name: one of the greenest cities in America (Penner 2013).

San Francisco, California, has passed a law requiring all new residential and commercial buildings of ten stories high or more to install solar panels to meet the building's heat and electrical needs (Sabatini 2016). The entire country of France now requires new buildings in commercial zones to have either solar panels or plants covering the rooftop (Agence France-Presse 2015).

Green rooftops bring multiple benefits. They improve air quality by reducing pollution particulates and carbon dioxide, removing heavy metals, and adding oxygen. They provide thermal insulation in both summer and winter, which lowers the building's overall energy consumption, and they also offer residents the advantage of sound insulation in urban areas. When designed with local plants, these rooftop environments support the natural biodiversity of the region, and the green aesthetics enhance emotional wellbeing and reduce stress (Sandler and David 2011).

RENEWABLES: TRANSPORTATION
AND ENERGY SOURCES

People worldwide are looking for ways to reduce fossil fuel use and lower their carbon footprint. In the transportation sector, electric bike sales have grown from 70,000 in 2012 to 270,000 in 2014 (*Yes! Magazine* 2016). Many urban areas are investing in bicycle infrastructure, including dedicated bike lanes that are not shared by cars, buses, or pedestrians (Colville-Andersen 2015).

The International Energy Agency reported that in 2015, 90 percent of all new energy capacity built globally was renewable (Werber 2016), and solar power has almost reached the goal of becoming as cost-effective as electricity (Thomas 2016). Denmark set a new world record for harnessing wind energy (Phillips 2015), and Australia, Ireland, Scotland, Germany, and the UK have also seen massive growth in renewables (Hall 2016; Smith 2015b).

PLANET-FRIENDLY FOOD PRODUCTION

Positive innovations in food production are rising out of increased awareness of the environmental costs of agro-business. One of the chief contributors to climate change is the leveling of jungles and forests to plant crops and graze cattle, which devastates habitat and causes species extinction, in addition to its impact on the global carbon cycle. Other destructive factors include the high carbon footprint of meat production, excessive food waste, transportation and the resulting pollution, pesticide use, unjust labor practices, and water overconsumption.

Groups that are supporting healthy ecosystems with community-based cooperative gardens, farmer's markets, and seed libraries are popping up everywhere. In the United States, Cleveland, Ohio, leads the way. In 2010, zoning regulations were altered to allow agriculture as a principal use on all vacant residential lots in the city. As a result, there are now more than 200 community gardens and urban farms in the city, and a recent study shows 1,108 more potential sites for urban agriculture there (Popovitch 2014; Schultz et al. 2014).

A neighborhood in Burderim, Australia, is designed around the principles of permaculture. Residents have planted garden rows along the streets in an 11-block stretch, resulting in an abundance of curbside fruits, vegetables, herbs, and spices. Neighbors are encouraged to take what they need as they collectively work to keep it thriving. In 2015, "Banana Boulevard" produced close to 2,000 pounds of fruit (Tatham and Gaffney 2016). Built on similar principles, in the city center of Seattle, Washington, is a seven-acre "food forest," with fruit-bearing trees and bushes where public foraging is encouraged (Husted 2012).

Many people are becoming more aware of the environmental cost of eating dairy and meat, particularly beef, and are eliminating or reducing their consumption. Scientists at the University of Oxford, in partnership with the Food and Agricultural Organization of the United Nations, released a study that confirms that a widespread transition to a vegetarian diet would cut carbon and methane emissions by nearly two-thirds (Fischer and Garnett 2016). In beef production there are multiple factors that contribute to environmental pollution, making beef "the new SUV" (Sutter 2015): there are issues of land use, pesticides, fertilizers, digestion-generated methane, and the fuel and water needed to produce feed for the animals.

Ecovillages

In addition to the urban areas that are designing greener policies and practices, there are thousands of rural ecovillages worldwide. These are intentional communities that take these cooperative efforts even further. One of the oldest is Sólheimar, located in southwest Iceland. It was founded in 1930 and is home to 100 residents who are striving to create a self-sustaining society based on the values of a creative work life, strong social ties, organic farming, and renewable energy. It has the only certified organic forestry sales center in Iceland, and the community works closely with the government and surrounding communities to offer environmental education, internships, and retreats (Fehrenbacher 2014).

Auroville in South India is the world's largest ecovillage. It got its start in 1968 and is currently home to 50,000 people from 49 countries. Organic horticulture is a core practice, and like many of these communities Auroville has a history of exploring new economic models. They began with a barter and exchange system, and there is still a large "free store" that, as the name implies, offers clothing, dishes, books, and music to community members at no cost, along with a free tailoring service (Thomas and Thomas 2013).

New economic models

A "gift economy" is also being explored at the corporate level in the United States, with Panera Bread opening "Panera Cares Cafes" in St. Louis, Detroit, and Portland. The dishes on the menu are offered "by donation," using a pay-what-you-can system. Panera's founder Ron Shaich reports that the pilot is going well, and he suggests that we should "Trust people—they'll surprise you" (Sher 2014, p.1).

"Open sourcing" is a concept that emerged in the field of computer technology; certain software source codes are made available to the general public for use and/or modification from the original design, rather than being controlled by a developer or corporation. This model is being expanded to industrialized production by physicist Marcin Jakubowski. He founded Open Source Ecology, which is home to Factor e Farm in Missouri. Jakubowski's goal is to create an open source blueprint of the 50 most important machines used in modern life—including an oven, a tractor, and a circuit—so that people can build and maintain their own machines at a fraction of what they would cost to purchase (Goodier 2011).

A NON-RESILIENT POLITICAL SYSTEM

Mark Jacobson and Mark Delucchi, two researchers based at Stanford University and the University of California, respectively, are ready to revolutionize the global adoption of renewable energy devices. They have spelled out in great detail how 139 nations can generate all the energy needed for homes, businesses, industry, transportation, and agriculture from wind, solar, and water power technologies by 2050. The plan emphasizes that the obstacles to implementing a 100 percent renewable global energy system are, "primarily social and political, not technological or even economic" (Jacobson and Delucchi 2011, p.1170). They assert the need for policymakers to, "Find ways to resist lobbying by the entrenched energy industries" (2009, p.4) and to provide strong leadership so that nations will respond to technologies vetted by scientists rather than promoted by corporations (2011).

Attempts to implement green programs on a large scale remind us of how complex and layered our climate issues are. As we have seen, they encompass everything from social justice, politics, education, and technology to the very evolution of human consciousness. Many innovative individual and community programs have been launched by the recognition of the urgent need for climate change action, but they have been frustrated by a sluggish response at policy levels. Human innovation has usually started at the margins and eventually become mainstream. Freewheeling creativity, by nature, arises from an innate awareness of realities not yet manifest.

As disheartening as our entrenched systems are, we can recall that there are many doorways through which we can participate in transformative change, and that there is a genuine need for people from all walks of life with a great range of skills to do the real work at hand. There is a powerful momentum building from many sectors to address our current condition.

Deep inquiry, compassion, and social capital

As we circle back to examining our potential contributions to resiliency in the mental health field, we can remember that engineers, organic farmers, politicians, and city planners, are all people, and that the quality of our relationships to ourselves, each other, and the environment remain at the heart of solutions to climate concerns. Once our compassionate connection to each other and the planet is awakened, the skills required will naturally flow into place.

Daniel Aldrich, Co-Director of Northeastern University's Security and Resilience Studies program, emphasizes that it is social capital, our connections to and caring for each other—not the money poured into infrastructure—that most quickly leads to recovery following a climate disaster. His data supports this perspective, regardless of the economic status of the community. He reports, "In communities of trust, fewer lives were lost. People who were healthy knew the people who were sick. They knocked on doors and said, 'Let's get out together'... You should be investing in the social infrastructure of a community" (English 2015, p.1). Yet today more than five times more money is invested in disaster responses than in disaster risk reduction (Jones 2016).

Psychology's call to action

There is much to do, and there is much we can do. At the time of completing this book, according to NASA no human alive had ever seen our earth as hot as it had been for the last seven sequential months (Plait 2016), with each high-temperature record shattering the previous one. By the first three months of 2016, the global temperature change averaged 1.48°C, essentially meeting the 1.5°C warming threshold defined by COP21 worldwide negotiators in Paris in December 2015 (Climate Central 2016). Science reported that the alarming trend of species decline is causing some researchers to question whether we have already surpassed the biodiversity limits required to support human life (Johnston 2016). Scientists with the National Oceanic and Atmospheric Administration reported that the level of carbon dioxide in the atmosphere in the Antarctic just reached a level that has not been seen in four million years (Kahn 2016). The key factors implicated in climate change are clearly not under control.

We need to recognize that the earth's living system—including the full range of diverse plant and animal life—is our true home. Understanding that our web of life is contained within a finite biosphere is essential. We can think of hope as a state of mind that, if paired with the right tools, can help us find our individual role in supporting a systemic, planet-healthy transformation.

Resiliency is encoded in our human genetics or we would not have made it this far. What if, as mental health professions, we join with other disciplines to support regenerative transformation in a number of ways, including:

- helping our clients process the full range of emotions triggered by climate chaos and helping them anchor their resiliency in order to act in alignment with their values

- supporting our clients to cultivate the deep connections required to build social capital, in order to balance the more superficial interactions promoted by our growing investment in social media

- creating a space for our clients to explore safely and open to life's challenges with courage and creativity

- reflecting back to our clients how valuable and unique their presence, voice, and contribution can be in shaping our world

- facilitating deep inquiry to help clients clarify their role and purpose, exploring with them unexamined beliefs that may get in their way of a regenerative orientation

- as in ecopsychology, encouraging our clients to experience a visceral and emotional connection with the natural world

- supporting clients to recognize that caring for the natural world is an investment in their own wellbeing

- helping individuals, couples, and communities build internal resilience that will stabilize their ability to function well in their respective fields

- treating the trauma, anxiety, depression, and self-doubt that interfere with a satisfying and engaged life

- cultivating creativity to promote out-of-the-box solutions and fresh perspectives

- teaching communication skills and supporting people to use their voice to share their experiences with others

- increasing tolerance for intense feelings, conflict, and disturbing situations

- assisting individuals to plan and undertake manageable shifts in behavioral patterns, and exploring resistance to change

- validating and normalizing grieving

- teaching self-care tools

- providing resources for additional forms of support

- modeling community involvement.

I know that some or all of these principles are already part of many psychotherapist's practices right now, so it will not be difficult to foster a professional frame of reference and defined competencies for the field of climate psychology within the mental health professions. Intake forms can be updated to add questions like, "Do you experience distress from current world events, including our changing climate?" They may be accompanied by a scale from "not at all" to "very distressed," with space to "describe your experience." Because all intake responses are reviewed with our clients, this approach can easily bring the conversation into the therapy room. We can raise awareness, hone our climate psychology assessment lens, expand our treatment skills, and have a more far-reaching influence. I recommend that this orientation and methodology enter into the required curriculum of psychotherapy training programs. Starting right now, we can make a conscious choice to make the effort to discover what will work and put more of our energy into what the world so deeply needs.

Additional resources

Aldrich, D. (2012) *Building Resilience: Social Capital in Post-Disaster Recovery.* Chicago, IL: University of Chicago Press.

Chalquist, C. (2007) *Terrapsychology: Reengaging the Soul of Place.* New Orleans, LA: Spring Journal Books.

Stiglitz, J. (2013) *The Price of Inequality: How Today's Divided Society Endangers Our Future.* New York, NY: WW Norton and Company.

Project Drawdown (2017) *Drawdown.* Sausalito, CA: Project Drawdown. More information is available at www.drawdown.org/the-book.

WORKSHEET

Listening to your heart and the heart of the earth

Close your eyes and sit in comfort and ease while remaining alert. Release your focus from the activities of your day and turn your attention to your breath. Become aware of the energy of your breath in your chest, in the area of your heart. When you inhale, expand your heart space, and with each exhale, relax and soften into it. Enjoy this process. Allow the energy of your breath to feed the openness of your heart.

Now invite an image to form in your expansive heart of the living earth. This image can appear in any way: as a vision of our planet, or some living being on the earth, or an abstract symbol. Be open to the way the image forms, even if it surprises you or doesn't make sense at first. Allow time for the vision to reside in your heart. As the image takes shape, notice everything about it: the color, texture, size. What qualities does it have? What is it saying right now? What does it want or need? Communication in imagery does not always occur in words—notice any impressions or a shift in qualities. Go ahead and respond to any messages or requests, knowing that with imagery many things are possible.

Continue in the presence of the living earth in your heart space. When this visioning feels complete for now, knowing that you can return at another time in a similar way, begin to gently find a closure, with gratitude, bringing your feelings and insights back into the room and opening your eyes.

Take time to write or draw your experiences and the actions you can take to honor your relationship to the earth.

Cultivating compassion—*Metta* or Lovingkindness Practice

There is not a single being more worthwhile of your kindness than yourself, although many of us struggle with feeling undeserving. Traditionally this practice begins with wishing well to oneself and then gradually expanding the kind wishes out to loved ones, friends, neighbors, acquaintances, strangers, eventually to people with whom you have difficulty, and ultimately to all beings.

Included here is an abbreviated three-step practice that includes our care for the earth.[1] When the issues of climate change get difficult, this is a practice that can hold both the joys and sorrows.

Take a few clearing breaths and connect again with your heart energy. The most important factor is to maintain your lovingkindness intention during the exercise. It is helpful to imagine yourself, another being, or the earth as you repeat the phrases. The first time through, use the word "I" in the four phrases. In the second repetition, choose a friend or loved one. The third time through, use the phrase "the living earth." There is no pressure to feel or experience anything in particular. However, if feelings of warmth or love arise, connect to these qualities as you continue. Mentally repeat, slowly and steadily, the following or similar phrases.

May _____ be happy and know joy.

May _____ be healthy and dwell in wellbeing.

May _____ be safe, protected from inner and outer harm.

May _____ be peaceful and in harmony with all life.

How might your life change if you practiced both of these meditations on a regular basis for six months? Take a moment to reflect and imagine, and then write about what you experience.

_____

_____

_____

_____

_____

_____

_____

_____

_____

_____

_____

Part II

Vitalization of an Ecoharmonious Life

Twelve Body, Heart/Mind, and World Wise Practices

All the rich information you have just learned about climate change is of little use unless it becomes a catalyst for comprehensive transformation. Psychology is not philosophy: it is a methodology for living a more fulfilling life. Climate psychology goes several steps further, by integrating our personal and collective fulfillment in harmony with the natural world.

The distress that is triggered by climate change events finds deep healing as we fully restore our relationships with all of life from a more awakened, interconnected perspective—including making wise, simple, everyday choices. *We have the freedom to choose to do things differently.* While climate solutions are also systemic, our daily life becomes part of the recovery, not just by shrinking our personal carbon footprint, but also by modeling a hopeful and manageable shift in attitude and behavior that can be witnessed in our personal and professional circles.

These 12 exercises are easy to do, yet they will lead to profound outcomes if practiced consistently and wholeheartedly. There are three sections for each exercise that provide instructions for taking fully embodied, clear-minded, openhearted, and no-nonsense steps toward ecoharmonious living. Ideally, I recommend that the practices be performed as part of a year-long commitment to transformation. Devote an entire month to each theme, practicing the same exercises daily. This in-depth focus allows the nuances to be revealed and the deeper values to become so intimately familiar that new habits will take root.

For example, the first practice, "The (Really) Big Picture," asks you to name three of your strengths. Naming the qualities you most identify with may be fairly easy for the first few days. After the first week, you may need to start peeling back the layers of who you are in order to reveal who you could become. Perhaps you will begin citing qualities that you know are within you, but they have been lying dormant. It is also possible to use any of these practices, singly or in combination, in individual and group work with clients.

Instructions

Allow at least 15 minutes for each practice, with approximately five minutes for each section: Body Wise, Heart/Mind Wise, and World Wise. While the Body Wise practices are gentle, modify any physical instructions to care for your body's needs. Body Wise begins with you standing, unless otherwise indicated, and the Heart/Mind and World Wise parts of the practice that follow can be done sitting. Feel free to modify any aspect of the instructions; always honoring what feels appropriate for you in the moment. All of the practices can be explored in depth, so if you happen to have more than 15 minutes, you are invited to linger...

1

The (Really) Big Picture

Body Wise

Stand with your feet about hip-distance apart, relaxed but upright with your knees slightly bent. Feel your weight distributed evenly in both feet. Bend your arms, resting your elbows lightly at your waist, forearms parallel to the floor with palms turned upward. Breathe in, as though you could draw the energy from the sky into your body though your palms and the top of your head while you gently straighten your legs. As you exhale, turn your palms downward, directing the flow of the breath down through your body, through your feet, connecting with the earth. Bend your knees slightly on the out-breath. Repeat this breath and movement cycle for three minutes, feeling yourself connecting to the sky and the earth. You can do this with your eyes open or closed.

Heart/Mind Wise

Just as there are no two snowflakes alike, realize there is only one you, with your unique constellation of qualities and gifts. Yet "being yourself" is a process. As adults we often acquire styles of coping that can obscure, rather than support, who we really are. As musician Miles Davis puts it,

"Man, sometimes it takes you a long time to sound like yourself" (Snodgrass 2002, p.5).

Name three of your particular strengths. Are you a good listener; do you have a knack for cooking or mechanics; are you loyal; are you an athlete; do you have a good sense of humor; are you inventive? These three good characteristics are part of what makes you the one and only you. Write these strengths down on a piece of paper.

1. _____

2. _____

3. _____

Pause, then name your strengths again, sensing your unique contribution to this world.

World Wise

How can one or more of the strengths you identified be part of climate change solutions? If you are a good writer, can you blog or write a letter to the editor of your local paper? If you excel at planning and organization, would you want to host an educational evening or a fundraiser for your favorite non-profit? If you bake, can you donate food to a gathering you value?

Write your plan, with a clear timeline.

2

Kindness

Body Wise

It is just as important to be able to say "no" as it is to say "yes" in life, depending on what healthy boundaries each situation warrants. But we sometimes say no to pure kindness and love. This can happen for a variety of reasons: we do not believe we deserve it; we do not recognize it; we are afraid. The focus of this practice is on saying yes to receiving unadulterated kindness and love.

Stand and let your weight rest evenly on both feet. Begin with the palms of your hands in front of you with bent elbows, as though you were going to push on a wall. Internally say the word "no," and imagine there are doors leading into your heart that are closed and latched shut. Now say "yes," extending your arms opens to the sides like you are welcoming an embrace. Breathe into your chest, expanding it and feeling the doors of your heart opening. Repeat the "yes" and "no" posture a few times, really noticing the difference.

While it is not the aim to use these postures out in the world, this practice helps us more clearly identify the felt-sense of being open and receptive or shut down and closed off. As we increase our ability to recognize our internal stance in a variety of situations, it gives us greater access to choosing a different response rather than reacting out of habit.

Heart/Mind Wise

Most of us were raised with messages of not being "good enough." Maybe our siblings did better in school or we excelled in a way that created tension at home. Or we believe that we are too chubby or too skinny; the one with the wrong kind of hair or skin; we were too loud or too quiet. The list of how we should look and behave is endless, and it changes depending on whom we talk to. As children, we absorbed those devaluing views of ourselves, and we hide the resulting beliefs under a cloak of shame in order to fit in and be accepted. We then carry these powerful misperceptions about ourselves into adult life. To make matters worse, we do not realize that other people are doing the same thing. So we compare our hidden internal wounds against the external facades of others: she is so successful in her career; look at their ideal relationship; he is so fit and attractive and I am frumpy. The conclusion: they have it together and I do not.

Now imagine back when you were a very young child: pure, loving, and playful as children naturally are. Even if you do not recall the details of your life, envision the bright spirit you came into the world with. Send a kind, compassionate breath to your very young self, the one who only wants to thrive in love. Know that your own original nature still resides in you.

World Wise

Choose one day this week to practice offering and receiving kindness. As you move through your normal routines, keep your eyes open to moments when you might offer a kind, simple, gesture: holding open a door for someone with arms loaded with shopping bags; smiling at a child; voicing genuine appreciation to someone. How do you feel when you are kind? Also notice the ways that kindness comes your way. Write about your experiences at the end of each day.

3

Grounding

Body Wise

Sit on a chair with your feet resting solidly on the floor or earth and your spine comfortably upright. Bring your attention to the soles of your feet, noticing the sensation of gentle contact with the floor. Consider how, for thousands of years, your ancestors have walked in close contact with the earth, often barefoot, and their attunement to the earth has been passed along to you in your genetic makeup. Imagine now that your feet have energetic roots like the deep root system of a tree. Let your sole-roots reach down deep into the rich, nourishing earth. Feel its nourishment rising through your roots into your legs, torso, arms, and head, like sap rising up the trunk of a tree. Rest in the earth's dynamic stability. Be nourished by the deep silence. Be at home in the support.

Heart/Mind Wise

Become aware of your strongest emotion in this moment. Is it primarily frustration, contentment, grief, happiness, anger, hope, fear, longing? This is only a partial list of the full and subtle range of our natural human emotions, so pause now and identify your most dominant feeling. Whatever emotion is present, know that it is a passing, temporary experience. Treat your emotion as a guest, a visitor passing through the home of your internal experience. Imagine it as a traveler. Let there be at least as much space around your emotion as we would have around ourselves when resting in a comfortable room. As the host of your internal home, you do not need to let this guest set up camp. You can acknowledge it while it pays you a visit, respect it, and let it express itself to you, but you do not need to feed or pamper it. Or, if you enjoy this particular guest's company, or if it has something to share with you, treat it to tea and offer an invitation to linger.

World Wise

There are symbolic and psychological aspects of grounding, and then there is the literal ground beneath our feet. Research reveals that healthy soil can help reverse global warming (Ohlson 2014)! There are many ways to live in alignment with healthy soil practices.

Food production and waste is a huge issue that we can all work to improve. More than a third of all of the food that's produced worldwide is not consumed, either because of spoilage during transit or because more affluent areas throw away unused food. In the United States, the agribusiness of producing food that ends up being thrown away generates more greenhouse gas emissions than most *entire countries* (Smith 2015c).

If you garden, do you compost and enrich the soil, mirroring the natural recycling that occurs in nature? If you are not a gardener, some communities have curbside composting, where food scraps can be added to yard waste bins, which is a tremendous improvement over adding them to landfills, which produce and emit methane. Minimizing waste can reduce greenhouse gas emissions in the United States by more than 36 percent (Platt *et al.* 2008). Choose restaurants that engage in these practices and that feature seasonal, locally grown, and organic food.

Write about one lifestyle change that you will commit to, starting today, that would nourish the living soil and reduce food waste.

4

Humor

Body Wise

Our moods are contagious, and we can transfer joy to others with our laughter. Yoga and *chi gong* can both include "laughing meditation," and the quickest way to learn is to attend a group and "catch it" from someone. Thanks to our World Wide Web, it is now easy to do. Watch one of these YouTube videos:

1. Laughing Meditation, 30 Days of Intent #6, Deepak Chopra, posted October 18, 2012 on the Chopra Well Channel.[1]

2. Contagious Subway Laughter, posted on October 15, 2012 by Steve Mac.[2]

3. Laughing in the Metro is best against Bad Mood, posted on May 1, 2009 by Jürgen Gschiel.[3]

Heart/Mind Wise

Did you hear the one about the Dalai Lama in New York? He approaches a hot dog vendor and says, "Make me one with everything." When the Dalai Lama receives his (vegan?) hot dog, he hands the vendor a $20 bill for the $5 hot dog. The Dalai Lama stands there with his hand out, looking confused and asks, "Where's my change?" "I thought you'd know," replies the vendor as he pockets the $20, "All change must come from within."

Humor and the freedom to be playful that we had as children are doorways to experiencing our state of natural joy and wholeness. This resiliency exercise will require you to send any internal judges on a vacation so you can enjoy yourself, be silly, and play!

You will need piece of plain paper and colored markers or a pen. If you have markers, choose a color that reminds you of a relaxed and happy mood. Now place your pen or marker in the center of the paper, holding the pen with your non-dominant hand (if you are right-handed, use your left hand.) Close your eyes and draw one of your favorite childhood memories. You do not even need to lift your pen from the paper. (Yes, it may look a lot like scribbles when you open your eyes in a few moments. That is great!) If you draw a road, let yourself remember the dirt and pebbles you saw. If you're drawing the sky, remember how the air smells and how the sun feels on your skin. Recall vividly the experience of fun, reliving what it felt like in your body, mind, and heart.

When you are finished, tape your drawing to the fridge for a week or so to remind yourself of your wild, wonderful inner child—who is still alive and well.

World Wise

While we cannot necessarily show up for work with crayons sticking out of our pockets, we can discover profound gifts when we bring a childlike, less-filtered way of viewing the world into our adult life. Young children seem to know how to "seize the day" with fewer conditions: in rain or sun, heat or chill, with shoes or barefoot, it is always the perfect time simply to engage with whatever life is presenting. A discarded can on the road signals the start of a game with friends; the neighborhood woods is a call to adventure.

Even in the serious business of climate change, there is a valuable resource to be found in lightness, humor, and play. They can free us from of our fixed frame of mind and provide opportunities to discover new insights and cultivate our creative prowess.

Look around you right now and see your environment as though you are viewing it for the very first time, as though your surroundings are an invitation to creative adventure. Look around you, aiming for the purity of perception common in children, supported by the maturity of your life experiences. Even if you are in a very familiar setting, notice the contours of the trees and other objects, their textures, the play of light and shadow, the feel of the air on your skin, the expression on someone's face. The birds, leaves, and insects have never been in the particular configuration they are in now, and they never will be again. This moment has never been experienced before. Be curious about the stories that accompany everything you see, remembering that they will always be bigger and deeper than what you already know.

With this more direct, spontaneous way of abiding in the moment, can you recognize beauty, even delight, right where you are? Notice if a lightness begins to emerge in your body, emotions, and mind, making it easier for life to provoke a spontaneous burst of laughter. One of the first things we do as infants is laugh, and, if we are lucky, it will be one of the last things we do. Regardless of the circumstances of your life, right here and right now, can you feel an unmitigated surge of life that just might reach your lips as a smile?

5

Love

Body Wise

Sit comfortably and bring your attention to the center of your chest. You can close your eyes or just let them have a soft downward focus.

Imagine a loving, warm fire glowing in your heart. It can help evoke the feeling to picture someone, or even an animal, that you feel a strong loving connection with. Take time to visualize them. Relax your shoulders and jaw. Let each breath fan the fire, allowing your heart energy to become strong, bright, and steady. See or sense all the colors and textures of your heart fire. Now imagine the warmth of your heart traveling down your arms and into the palms of your hands.

Let the loving energy expand outward, up to the top of your head and down into your torso. Let your heart's embrace travel down your legs to the soles of your feet.

Now feel a full-bodied, openhearted glow, a radiant and loving halo within and around your whole body.

Heart/Mind Wise

Unfortunately, many of us did not experience consistent and supportive love at home as we were growing up. Even if we did receive what psychology would deem "good enough" parenting, as adults there continues to be a deep longing for being seen for who we are and being accepted as loveable, just as we are.

Using your paper and pen, write a letter to yourself that expresses things you wish you would have heard, or heard more often, from your primary caregivers. The letter can be free-form or you can use the template below. Go with your first impressions—it does not have to be long or a finished product.

Dear (Your Name),

I so appreciate the ways you _____ .

I delight in your _____ .

I am so sorry that I _____ .

I will always delight in your remarkable _____ .

May you flourish in your life, with loving relationships, fulfilling work, and joyous wellbeing.

Love always, _____

Now read the letter again to yourself, knowing that it is a mirror of the beautiful person that you are. Be like a sponge, taking in the love that is yours.

World Wise

Look around you and consider that life loves itself by becoming the myriad of forms it takes. Life loves itself by living through you. Life loves itself by living through all beings. But we are learning that not all actions reflect love and respect for life.

In Chapter 6 we read about human slavery in the Thai shrimp market and the abuse of workers in brand-name clothing factories. Take interest in and learn more about the story behind your food and other purchases. Take an inventory of the things in your kitchen, closet, and living room. After the survey, list three things you will now do/buy differently that are more ecoharmonious. Consider the changes not as a sacrifice, but as an act of love.

Record your change commitments on paper.

6

The Pulse of Life

Body Wise

Sit or recline comfortably and place the palm of your right hand over your heart, resting your left hand on top of the right. Feel or imagine the rhythm of your heartbeat. Close your eyes and sense your pulse. Your heartbeat was shared with your mother's, and it was transferred to you like a flame carried from one candle to another. Even if you had a difficult relationship with your mother, or did not know her, she still gave you the gift of life. Your mother's heartbeat was ignited by her mother, which was passed on from *her* mother. And so it goes on—a single heartbeat flowing through generations. Sense your connection to your ancestors, whether personally known to you or not. Continue to follow the steady rhythm further and further back in time. Feel the enduring river of life that now courses through your veins. Let your fingertips begin to lightly tap the beat of your heart on your chest, and rest in the soothing rhythm.

Heart/Mind Wise

It is estimated that the average number of heartbeats in a lifetime is slightly over two billion. While this is ultimately an unknown, how many beats might you have felt so far?

While the finite nature of our heartbeats is mysterious, and to acknowledge our mortality can even be frightening at times, it also contains a paradoxical invitation to a deeper life.

In my work in hospitals over the years, I have seen so many people who faced a life-threatening diagnosis who then discovered a radical call to life. By squarely facing the inevitability of death, life becomes so precious and valuable. Each day becomes heightened with gratitude and possibility.

But it does not require illness or tragedy to seize the invitation to live our lives fully. Pause and consider the gift of today. It arrives without guarantees of another. This day appears without our effort or earnings: it truly is a gift. Life brought you here; life is sustaining you; life will call you home. Take a moment to feel life as your universal mother, and like a child resting in the rhythm of its mother's heartbeat, let yourself rest in the rhythm of life itself.

Choose one thing, right now, in honor of the gift of this day: call a friend and tell them you appreciate them; enjoy the taste of a peach; sing; let go of self-criticism… As the saying goes, "If not now, when?"

World Wise

Things also have their lifecycle. Upcycling is a process of transforming unwanted items into something useful or beautiful, rather than discarding or recycling them. It helps create a circular economy by extending the lifespan of materials. We can bring our creativity to make this trash-to-treasure cycle elegant, rustic, or shabby-chic. Reducing waste is of tremendous benefit to the environment, and upcycling can also save us money!

As we change our consumer habits in an earth-friendly way, the possibilities are as boundless as your imagination. It can be fun to design new uses for things: for example, lining up a row of empty jars and planting a kitchen-counter herb garden, or turning an old picture frame into a serving tray. I have even seen old leather suitcases stacked to make a fun, vintage end-table.

The next time you walk toward the trash, recycle bin, or donation bag, pause and consider if you can see a hidden value in the object in your hand.

7

Garden State

Body Wise

Walk—around your land, your neighborhood, your city. Let it be a walking meditation, where you feel with heightened awareness the physical sensation of each step. Notice how much life wants to thrive: plants that insist on growing in the tiniest crack in the cement, flowers that seed an entire meadow and set a hillside ablaze with color.

Look closely to spy the blush hidden on the innermost petal of a flower; zoom out and see the complex contours and textures in an area where a variety of trees, bushes, and plants are thriving in their communal ecosystem. What do you smell, hear, and feel?

When you walk at different times of the year, notice the particular beauty of each season. Autumn gives us the rustle of leaves as they change and descend, blanketing the ground with a patchwork of yellow, orange, red, and brown. In winter the starkly elegant branches hold an invisible secret: they are protecting the green and blossoming promise of a time to come. The snow quiets everything down; manicured yards and overgrown fields look equally beautiful cloaked in white.

What else do you notice?

Heart/Mind Wise

Gardens can teach us much about ourselves and life. Plants will not grow any faster than nature determines, but we can help create the conditions that will encourage them to thrive. What conditions would best support your personal growth? Gardening is a practice that requires understanding, observation, consistent care, and patience. What better guidelines for our own unfolding.

Skillful gardening needs an understanding of context: plants that love the tropics will wither in the desert and vice versa. It helps to have the right tools. When we are wondering, "Will they ever grow?!" we might be tempted to dig into the soil to see if the seeds are sprouting, which is likely to damage the tender shoots. And what is our reaction when we hit a rocky patch?

There is a rhythm and cycle: preparing the soil, planting, weeding, nourishing, harvesting, and pruning. There is an interdependent relationship between the weather, soil type, insects, and other plants. We can see resiliency as we observe the trees that bend but do not break in the storm, and the return of spring.

What is the state of your mind and heart's garden? Do you have the right tools to thrive? Are your thoughts nourishing or toxic? Is it time to weed or to pause and enjoy the blossoming beauty?

Write about it.

World Wise

Would you consider converting your lawn into a garden? Becoming a guerilla gardener? Joining a community garden? Supporting or starting a seed library? Planting tomatoes or herbs in a pot? Volunteering at a local school that has a garden for their kids? Funding the planting of trees to restore deforestation?

Move from noticing and appreciating to becoming an active steward of life. As with all of these practices, it is less about following the suggestions listed here and more about launching your own ways of becoming engaged that are relevant to your life and local ecosystem. Notice what tugs on your heart, sparks your creativity—and then follow through.

Identify a step you can take, with a clear timeline, and write about it.

8

Who's Driving the Bus?

Heart/Mind Wise

Yes, you are right: we are switching the sequence this time, with the Body Wise practice following this reflection.

How is it that the person we were at 8:00 am, who so earnestly resolved to take a walk after work, does not seem like the same one who drove home at 5:00 pm and flipped on the TV? Who is in the driver's seat as these decisions are made? The practices in this book are about change, and understanding our own inner constitution goes a long way toward being successful at fulfilling our intentions.

We think of ourselves as a single, unified self, but it may be more helpful to become familiar with our multiple selves, or "subpersonalities," as we make sense of our lives. Popular psychology has acquainted us with the notion of an inner child, which is one type of subpersonality, but there is a wide range of others who make up our self's "team." Other common subpersonalities include the inner critic, the clown, the righteous one, the victim, the caretaker, the wise wo/man, the tyrant, the leader, the "I can't" naysayer. We all have a diverse collection of selves, and the specific constellation is unique to each person. The strength and dominance of each subpersonality is shaped by our life experiences, temperament, and mental habits—and they can change over time. Stressful moments can call out our more primitive subpersonalities, which may not best serve the situation at hand.

If you find you are not making the changes you hope for, you may want to check and see who has grabbed the steering wheel, and ask yourself if there is another part of you that can come forward and take the driver's seat.

Who is behind the wheel right now?

Body Wise

Think of a recent situation when you were of "two minds" about something, like our friend who was confident about taking that evening walk but ended up in front of the TV.

Find a posture that reflects your confident and healthy intention, letting your body express the strength of your desire. Maybe your hands are on your hips or your arms are outstretched. Try a few different positions until you find the one that feels most accurate. Now amplify it, exaggerating the posture. Really notice how you feel in your body, mind, and emotions.

Now find a posture that fully reflects the unintended outcome, your version of the TV instead of the walk, taking a full minute to experience this position, including an amplified version.

Go back and forth between the postures a few times, ending with a position that best reflects your healthy intention.

Because our physiology reacts along with our thoughts and feelings, our bodies can help us shift into our desired behavior. The next time you find yourself veering from your intention, try stepping into the posture of that intention for a full minute, and notice how it changes your experience.

World Wise

Just like we can "try on" a desired intention with a posture, we can also try on a way of being by acting "as if" it were already so. Psychologist Alfred Adler (2014) created an "as if" technique that encourages people to try acting *as if* they were already the person they aspire to be. For example, someone who wants to be "self-assured and outgoing" would begin to act out those qualities in daily situations. Start by practicing in low-risk settings, like the checkout line at a grocery store or in brief interactions with strangers. This is one way of rehearsing, and artists and athletes all know that practice is not just a wish to perform well, it also optimizes our performance by building neural pathways that fire up reliably in the midst of the stress of the real event. Rehearsing is one of the best ways to connect to our emotions and imagination.

What quality do you want to embody that would support you in engaging in environment-friendly actions?

Pick three times or situations when you will act "as if" you have already grown fully into that attribute, and write about the results.

9

The Stretch Zone

Body Wise

While this is a very gentle stretching exercise, be sure to respect your body's safe range of motion and modify if needed. Consult with your medical professional regarding movement restrictions.

As we stretch our bodies, stress is released and we gradually increase our range and fluidity of motion, along with ease in our minds and emotions. As you experience the movements, become even more aware of being present in your body.

Sit in a straight-backed chair with your feet resting on the floor and your spine upright. It is essential to move slowly and really feel into the physical sensations that accompany each movement. Repeat each instruction three to five times.

- Begin by closing your eyes and noting how your body feels: the level of fatigue, the degree of tension or relaxation, any areas of discomfort, and overall body presence.

- Open your eyes and scrunch your nose, lips, and eyebrows into a tight bunch in the center of your face. Then stretch your face as large as you can, opening your mouth, sticking out your tongue, and turning your eyes upward.

- Gently drop your chin toward your chest, letting it be heavy but keeping your torso upright. Roll your head to the right until your right ear is over your right shoulder. Then return your chin to your chest and roll to the left side.

- Lift your shoulders up to your ears with an in-breath, and let them drop down again with the exhalation.

- Make small forward circles with both shoulders, then reverse the direction.

- Place your fingertips on top of your shoulders, and draw circles with your elbows. Go both directions.

- With your arms down by your sides, gently shake your arms and hands.

- Gently twist your shoulders and upper torso to the right, looking over your right shoulder. Your hips remain facing forward. Repeat to the left.

- Extend your right leg a few inches off the ground and circle your ankle in both directions. Repeat on the other side.

- With both feet on the ground, alternately lift and drop just your heels in rapid succession, letting the vibrations travel up your body.

- Close your eyes and notice any changes in how you feel.

Heart/Mind Wise

To continue growing and developing, we need to move out of our comfort zone and into our stretch zone (without moving into our panic zone!). As we stretch our attitudes and behaviors, it also lowers our ambient stress over the long-term and gradually increases our range of options.

You can think of your familiar habits, skills, and knowledge as your comfort zone, and to stretch beyond that is to move into a learning zone. The edges of each zone are different for each person, and you will be the one to determine whether a new perspective or behavior is at the right level of challenge. In the stretch zone we can feel uncomfortable or vulnerable, but it also offers us an invitation for growth, exploration, and a chance to experiment. If you are reserved or introverted by nature, it might be a considerable stretch to speak up around others. If you are outgoing, the stretch could mean listening more attentively.

When it comes to responding to climate change concerns, where do you get stuck and where do you need to stretch? Can one of the "selves" we explored in the previous exercise be of help? Write the answers down.

World Wise

With climate change issues, time could not be more pressing. Moving into our stretch zone is one way to respond more quickly with our energy and talents. Is there a climate change action you value but have been avoiding, because it causes you some discomfort? The tension could be signaling an opportunity for you to stretch. Write about it now, and include an action plan.

10

Seeing Clearly

Body Wise

We have learned from science that the oxygen we take in with each breath nourishes every cell in our body. Taking a full but natural breath, imagine vitality and oxygen flowing upward, bringing clarity into your mind. Exhale, directing your breath down through your body from head to toe, releasing tension along the way. Direct the next inhalation to your heart, sending a comforting breath to ease any emotional tension. Exhale down the body again. Continue the breathe cycle for three minutes, continuing to relax your body as you clear your mind and soothe your heart with each breath.

Heart/Mind Wise

Anaïs Nin reminds us that, "We do not see things as they are, we see them as we are" (Nin 1972, p.124). Seeing the world as we are is tricky business, and it reveals why life gets so confusing and difficult at times. We become convinced that our perception of a person or situation is accurate, when we may not only be mistaken, we may also be completely unaware of how our view is based on our own unconscious and faulty assumptions.

Neuroscientists are revealing the culprit behind these mistaken impressions in what they call implicit memory. You can think of implicit memories as fragments of experience that are stored below the level of conscious awareness, and they make no distinction between past and present time. For example, if you were stung by a bee at three months of age, you likely do not have an explicit (conscious) memory of the event or how the people around you coped with it. There are many ways that this stored experience could be impacting your life today. You could be jumpy around buzzing insects, even harmless ones, without knowing why. Or if you were in a big crowd when you were stung, you may have associated the pain with a closed-in feeling, and now you are a bit claustrophobic. It might have become a piece of evidence in a belief system that the world is a dangerous place, especially if this belief has been bolstered by other experiences that all ended up deepening the same neural grooves. So things that feel like our intuition or gut reaction may only be a distorted reenactment of an implicit memory.

One indication that implicit memories may be racing down our neural pathways is when our reaction is bigger than the situation warrants, even though our reactions will feel completely justified in the moment. It is usually in retrospect that we realize we were hijacked by intense emotions and overreacted. These "bigger" reactions can take many forms, including an angry outburst, tearful withdrawal, or stunned, bewildering confusion.

The good news is that we are not at the mercy of our neural programming or even stuck with our particular temperament. We can modify our reactions, calm the amygdala's instincts, and create new neural pathways when we intentionally engage our prefrontal cortex. The prefrontal cortex manages the amygdala's emotions, gleaning their valuable messages and then integrating thoughts and feelings in a flexible and discerning way.

World Wise

The next time you find yourself having an outsized emotional reaction, take a few breaths and allow the feelings to ease in your body, and then begin to examine your mental commentary. While some of the injustice and suffering related to climate change truly warrants a strong response, if we remain in an emotionally inflamed state it serves no one, including ourselves. Notice if climate events involving loss, trauma, or suffering are triggering any earlier personal experiences, and know that climate change work requires healing on both the personal and global levels. With awareness, channel your appropriate, righteous outrage into corrective climate action, such as: supporting policy change; entering into the social discourse; climate art; initiating or signing petitions; attending peaceful protests; and educating yourself and others. Be specific: what steps can you take in the upcoming month?

11

One Body

Body Wise

Notice your breath. At what point does it change from being the *air around you* to becoming *your breath*—when it enters your body at the tip of your nose, halfway into your nasal passage, when it fills your lungs?

When does the *air around you* stop being the *sky*—when you are in a room? What if the doors and windows are open? When does the *sky* stop being the *space* that stretches throughout the universe? Consider that the *sky* becomes a *part of you* as the oxygen molecules travel to every cell in your body.

For several minutes, bring awareness to your breath as you release the words that create the separation between breath, air, and sky. Experience the edgeless living breath, the same one breathed by all beings. Now simply relax and allow yourself to "be breathed" by life.

Heart/Mind Wise

Did you know that each carbon atom in our bodies was once blasted from a star? With science confirming that we are indeed stardust, perhaps it becomes a little less clear where we stop and start and the rest of the universe begins. While words are convenient when it comes to asking for salt at the dinner table, and the edges of the cup are handy for knowing where to pour the tea, when we only function in an object-oriented world, without connecting to the overarching connectedness of life, we are desensitized to the world's vitality and we overemphasize separation— which, as we have seen, is a core contributor to climate change. Not only does this limited perspective contribute to a life out of balance, it also robs us of some of the most basic wonders of our human experience.

How might we move toward a visceral knowing that the forest is part of our lungs, the rivers part of our circulation? This is not just poetic imagery; it literally cannot be more realistic and practical.

World Wise

It is possible, even essential, to unite *doing* and *being* as one experience, one practice. We can make simple daily choices with the awareness that they arise from, return to, and are part of the web of life. We have taken time to look at where our food and various everyday items originate. Now let us now understand more about where things go.

We know that tons of plastic end up in the ocean, and 40 million Americans are ingesting pharmaceuticals in contaminated drinking water (Scheer and Moss 2011). As we reduce our consumption, we can also take time to research the most planet-friendly options for waste disposal in our area, knowing that, in the words of Dkhw'Duw'Absh Chief Seattle, "Whatever we do to the web (of life), we do to ourselves" (Hernandez-Wolfe 2013, p.107). After you have reduced waste, composted, recycled, and upcycled, record here what you discovered about the healthiest waste disposal options in your community. If you need a little inspiration and some tips, look up Lauren Singer, a real shining star in the zero-waste movement: she fitted four years of trash into a 16-ounce Mason jar (East 2016).

12

Gratitude

Body Wise

While all of us are in varying states of health, we are still here because a good portion of our bodies are working well. Begin in a comfortable sitting or reclining position, with your eyes closed or softly gazing downward.

Bring your awareness into your feet and legs, and consider all the ways that they have taken you where you needed or wanted to go. Send a breath of appreciation into your legs.

Now focus on your torso, your strong and flexible spine, the numerous organs working beautifully together. Can you feel the beating of your heart? Notice the movement of your breath. Consider the ways your vital organs transform nutrition into energy for your work and enjoyment. Breathe appreciation into the muscles, bones, and organs of your torso.

Bring your awareness into your arms and hands, and remember all the things they touch and hold. Give back to them for a moment, with a breath of gratitude.

As your eyes rest, consider all the ways they take in the world, and the sounds your ears register, and your senses of taste, smell, and touch. They help keep us safe and make the world come alive in our interactions. Nourish all your sense organs with your breath as you acknowledge all that they do. And that brain of yours—you would not want to be without one! Infuse your mind and brain with gratitude.

Remaining in a state of gratitude, when you are ready open your eyes again.

Heart/Mind Wise

Chuang Tzu, the Taoist sage from the fourth-century B.C., is believed to have said that in every moment there are 10,000 joys and 10,000 sorrows (Bernhard 2013). But based on how our brains process information, we tend to remember the negative events at a ratio of five to one (Baumeister *et al.* 2001), so it often feels as though there are 10,000 joys and 50,000 sorrows. Gratitude is a wonderful way to bring our perceptions back into balance, and it is a choice we can make.

Gratitude is derived from the same linguistic roots—gratus, grata, or gratia—as the word grace (Pohl 2012), meaning a gift that is freely given or unearned. To cultivate gratitude, we can create a new habit of noticing the positive things that come our way. We can appreciate when we do *not* have a toothache or backache and enjoy more and more the stabilizing and healing properties of gratitude.

What is right in your life at this time? Write down a few things now.

World Wise

If you recorded just ten moments from your day that you were grateful for, in less than three years you would have named more than 10,000 joys. While there is no need to be exacting about the number, practice noticing what is good on a daily basis, as you feel and express gratitude for what is working in your life.

Gratitude is not just a "feel-good" activity, although it does make you feel good! When cultivated, research has shown that it has a host of benefits, including boosting the immune system, improving sleep, lowering blood pressure, reducing pain, diminishing isolation, and increasing alertness (Emmons 2010). Like so many of the resiliency exercises in these pages, practicing gratitude alters neural pathways, which makes the feelings and attitudes it invokes easier to sustain over time and become a more consistent inclination (Kini *et al.* 2016).

As a part of climate change work, gratitude not only builds our inner moxie when we encounter tough situations and emotions run high, it's also one of the innate qualities that naturally arise when we truly recognize our deep connection with the natural world.

Thank the people at the forefront of climate change movements, the innovators, activists, educators, and political leaders who are compassionately fierce in their efforts. Thank your friends, colleagues, and neighbors for the green actions you witness them supporting in everyday life. Thank yourself for having the courage to show up and make changes. The more we collectively embody gratitude, the sooner we will create the world we can imagine for ourselves and for generations to come. In the words of the poet Mary Oliver, "Of course! The path to heaven doesn't lie down in flat miles. It's in the imagination with which you perceive this world, and the gestures with which you honor it" (Oliver 1992, p.79).

Appendix

PROGRESSIVE RELAXATION[1]

Find a place to sit comfortably, or recline, as long as you can be relaxed but remain alert for this exercise. If you can, loosen tight or restrictive clothing. Allow yourself 20 minutes of undisturbed time.

Close your eyes, or allow them to have a soft, downward focus. Take three clearing breaths, welcoming in the oxygen and fresh energy with as much ease as possible. Each time you breathe out, let the breath begin to rinse stress and tension from your body. Imagine the breath circulating up to the top of your head, and down to the soles of your feet: full body breathing.

Now become aware of all the areas of contact between your body and the chair, cushions, or floor. Let those sensations be a signal to relax, letting those parts of your body receive the support. Each time you exhale, let yourself relax a little more deeply, as though you could release worry and tension with each exhalation. Each time you breathe in, note the refreshing quality of a new breath. Let it be easy—just let the relaxation happen. Know that your body enjoys relaxing, and it will do so naturally if you let it.

Bring your awareness to the top of your head, and notice any sensations along your scalp and forehead. If at any time you feel tightness or holding that is not useful, explore softening those areas as you exhale. Continue by bringing your attention to your face, letting your eyes rest and your jaw be loose and slack. Send a breath to your neck, shoulders, and upper back, deepening the relaxation as you exhale. Allow any accumulated stress slip off your shoulders like taking off a heavy winter coat. Let the relaxation flow into both arms, hands, and fingers, like a gentle internal breeze. Let your awareness travel throughout your torso, infusing the vital organs with fresh oxygen as you breathe in, and relaxing as you breathe out. Continue relaxing into your hips and legs, letting your breath flow down into the soles of your feet and your toes.

As you relax, it allows your body's natural healing abilities to work optimally, without being told what to do. Feel or imagine your deep reserves of wellbeing.

As you continue to relax, turn your attention to your mind, noticing that your mind is different than your thoughts. The mind is like a sky, or a vast field of awareness, through which your thoughts travel. Let your thoughts be like birds that fly through the sky. For the next few moments, when you become aware of any thoughts, treat them all the same, whether it is a memory, a detail, a worry, or plan—just let them be different kinds of birds. You do not need to chase them off or feed them. They will be present for a time and then continue on their way.

See if you can become even more aware of the spaces between your thoughts, and around your thoughts. Notice, even if it is just a flash of awareness, how the sky-like mind is peaceful.

When you let thoughts pass by, it helps the body relax. As you relax your body, it helps create space between your thoughts.

If at any time, you notice yourself becoming distracted, just take another full breath and gently return your attention to this practice. Give yourself a few moments to enjoy the relaxation and benefit from the comfort that will support you in all aspects of your life. You may be surprised to discover you return to doing whatever you need to accomplish with greater ease than you thought was possible.

Now bring your awareness to your emotions, wherever you sense that part of yourself. In the same way you have extended an invitation to your body and mind to relax, you can do the same with your emotions. Without requiring that anything in particular happen, just know that this is a good time for resting. Bring kind acceptance to whatever you are experiencing.

And now move your awareness even more deeply inside yourself, deeper than the fluctuating body sensations, deeper than the coming and going of thoughts and feelings, to the energy that animates you: a core vitality, an aliveness, a quality of wellbeing that infuses all the levels of who you are.

Rest now in a three-dimensional awareness of being present in your body, with a spacious mind and open heart, connected to the source that animates all of life. Let it be easy. Just rest in the awareness.

*As we prepare to bring this to a close, notice any shifts that you have found valuable or important during this practice; let the benefits imprint themselves in you so that your body remembers the feelings, along with your mind and heart.

Remain connected to any useful shifts while you begin to sense the room around you again. Notice once more the areas of contact with the cushions or floor; feel the ebb and flow of your breath; notice the temperature of the air on your skin; and register any sounds you can hear. As you are ready, fully present in your body with relaxation and ease, gradually open your eyes.

---

*   If this is a preparation for the Remembered Strength or Peaceful Place exercise, skip these closing paragraphs and move directly into the other script.

REFERENCES

350.org (2016) "Homepage." Available at http://350.org, accessed on 23 August 2016.

Adler, A. (2014) *The Practice and Theory of Individual Psychology.* Bensenville, IL: Lushena Books.

Agence France-Presse (2015) "France decrees new rooftops must be covered in plants or solar panels." *The Guardian*, 20 March 2015. Available at www.theguardian. com/world/2015/mar/20/france-decrees-new-rooftops-must-be-covered-in-plants-or-solar-panels, accessed on 25 August 2016.

Aguilar, J. (2015) "Two years later, 2013 Colorado floods remain a 'nightmare' for some." *The Denver Post*, 12 September 2015. Available at www.denverpost. com/2015/09/12/two-years-later-2013-colorado-floods-remain-a-nightmare-for-some, accessed on 25 August 2016.

Ainsworth, M. D. S. (1973) "The development of infant-mother attachment." *Review of Child Development Research 3*, 1–94.

Aldern, C. (2016) "Mountaintop removal country's mental health crisis." *Grist.* Available at http://grist.org/climate-energy/mountaintop-removal-countrys-mental-health-crisis, accessed on 25 August 2016.

Andrews, G. (2012) "Plastics in the ocean affecting human health." *Geology and Human Health, National Association of Geoscience Teachers.* Available at http://serc.carleton.edu/NAGTWorkshops/health/case_studies/plastics.html, accessed on 25 August 2016.

Arrien, A. (2014) "Cornerstones of wisdom: the four-fold way." *TEDxFiDiWomen.* Available at www.youtube.com/watch?v=2kDRRBK95no, accessed on 25 August 2016.

Aston, C. (2014) "Retrospective: disaster response." *Shambhala Times.* http://shambhalatimes.org/2014/10/10/retrospective-disaster-response, accessed on 25 August 2016.

Azar, B. (2000) "A new stress paradigm for women." *American Psychological Association, Monitor on Psychology 31*, 7, 42.

Baer, R. (2003) "Mindfulness training as a clinical intervention: a conceptual and empirical review." *Clinical Psychology: Science and Practice 10*, 125–143.

Balaban, V., Becker, W., Bourne, P., Bray, J. *et al.* (2012) *The Psychological Effects of Global Warming on the United States.* Available at www.nwf.org/pdf/Reports/ Psych_Effects_Climate_Change_Full_3_23.pdf, accessed on 25 August 2016.

Balbus, J., Crimmins, A., Gamble, J., Easterling, D. *et al.* (2016) "Climate change and human health." In: Balbus, J., Crimmins, A., Gamble, J., Easterling, D. *et al.* (2016) *The Impacts of Climate Change on Human Health in the United States: A Scientific Assessment*, 25–42.

Baldwin, J. (2011) *The Cross of Redemption: Uncollected Writings.* New York, NY: Vintage Books/Random House.

Baumeister, R., Bratslavsky, E., Finkenauer, C., and Vohs, K. D. (2001) "Bad is stronger than good." *Review of General Psychology 5*, 323–370.

Bava, S., Pulleyblank Coffey, E., Weingarten, K., and Becker, C. (2010) "Lessons in collaboration, four years post-Katrina." *Family Process 49*, 4, 543–558.

Bazerman, M. H., Baron, J., and Shonk, K. (2001) *You Can't Enlarge the Pie: Six Barriers to Effective Government.* New York, NY: Basic Books.

Bechtel, R. and Churchman, A. (2002) *Handbook of Environmental Psychology.* New York, NY: Wiley.

Bell, P., Greene, T., Fisher, J., and Baum, A. (2001) *Environmental Psychology.* Fort Worth, TX: Harcourt College Publishers.

Bernhard, T. (2013) *How to Wake Up: A Buddhist-Inspired Guide to Navigating Joy and Sorrow.* Somerville, MA: Wisdom Publications.

Bernstein, A. and Rice, M. (2013) "Lungs in a warming world: climate change and respiratory health." *Chest 143*, 5, 1455–1459.

Berry, T. (1999) *The Great Work: Our Way into the Future.* New York, NY: Bell Tower.

Betancourt, T., Speelman, L., Onyango, G., and Bolton, P. (2009) "A qualitative study of mental health problems among children displaced by war in northern Uganda." *Transcultural Psychiatry 46*, 2, 238–256.

Bienick, D. (2016) "Water boil advisory lifted for Sacramento's Pocket area." *KCRA News.* Available at www.kcra.com/news/local-news/news-sacramento/ voluntary-boil-advisory-issued-for-parts-of-sacramento/37368372, accessed on 25 August 2016.

Bill, J. and Chavez, R. (2002) "The politics of incoherence: the United States and the Middle East." *Middle East Journal 56*, 4, 562–575.

Blakemore, B. (2006) "Category 6 hurricanes? They've happened." *ABC News.* Available at http://abcnews.go.com/GMA/Science/story?id=1986862, accessed on 25 August 2016.

Boeskool, C. (2016) "When you're accustomed to privilege, equality feels like oppression." *Huffington Post.* Available at www.huffingtonpost.com/chris-boeskool/when-youre-accustomed-to-privilege_b_9460662.html, accessed on 25 August 2016.

Bowlby J. (1983) *Attachment: Attachment and Loss, Volume One*. New York, NY: Basic Books.

Brock, R. and Lettini, G. (2013) *Soul Repair: Recovering from Moral Injury after War*. Boston, MA: Beacon Press.

Brouillette, R. (2016) "Why therapists should talk politics." *The New York Times*. Available at http://opinionator.blogs.nytimes.com/2016/03/15/why-therapists-should-talk-politics/?_r=1, accessed on 25 August 2016.

Brown, J. and Isaacs, D. (2005) *The World Café: Shaping our Futures Through Conversations that Matter*. San Francisco, CA: Berrett-Koehler Publishers, Inc.

Brown, M. E., Antle, J. M., Backlund, P., Carr, E. R. *et al*. (2015) "Climate change, global food security, and the U.S. food system." *U.S. Department of Agriculture, the University Corporation for Atmospheric Research, and the National Center for Atmospheric Research*. Available at www.usda.gov/oce/climate_change/ FoodSecurity2015Assessment/FullAssessment.pdf, accessed on 25 August 2016.

Brumfiel, G. (2013) "Fukushima: fallout of fear." *Nature*, 16 January 2013. Available at www.nature.com/news/fukushima-fallout-of-fear-1.12194, accessed on 25 August 2016.

Campbell, J. (2016) "Are we raising a generation of nature-phobic kids?" *Los Angeles Times*, 29 July 2016. Available at www.latimes.com/opinion/op-ed/la-oe-campbell-kids-fear-of-nature-20160729-snap-story.html, accessed on 25 August 2016.

Campbell, J. and Osbon, D. (1995) *Reflections on the Art of Living: A Joseph Campbell Companion*. New York, NY: HarperCollins.

Campbell, T. and Kay, A. (2014) "Solution aversion: on the relation between ideology and motivated disbelief." *Journal of Personality and Social Psychology 107*, 5, 809–824.

Chemtob, C., Tomas, S., Law, W., and Cremniter, D. (1997) "Post disaster psychosocial intervention." *American Journal of Psychiatry 154*, 415–417.

Chödrön, P. (2001) *Start Where You Are: A Guide to Compassionate Living*. Boston, MA: Shambhala Publications, Inc.

Christ, C. (2016) "As the world sinks." *National Geographic Traveler*. Available at http://travel.nationalgeographic.com/travel/traveler-magazine/tales-from-the-frontier/maldives, accessed on 25 August 2016.

Climate Central (2016) "Earth flirts with a 1.5 degree Celsius global warming threshold." *Scientific American*, 20 April 2016. Available at www.scientificamerican.com/ article/earth-flirts-with-a-1-5-degree-celsius-global-warming-threshold1, accessed on 25 August 2016.

Clinton County Health Department (2016) "Boil water orders." *Clinton County Health Department*. Available at www.clintonhealth.org/bwo, accessed on 25 August 2016.

Cohen, K. (2006) *Honoring the Medicine: The Essential Guide to Native American Healing*. New York, NY: Ballantine Books.

Colville-Andersen, M. (2015) "The 20 most bike-friendly cities on the planet." *Wired*. Available at www.wired.com/2015/06/copenhagenize-worlds-most-bike-friendly-cities, accessed on 25 August 2016.

Confino, J. (2016) "This Buddhist monk is an unsung hero in the world's climate fight." *Huffington Post World Economic Forum*, 22 January 2016. Available at www.huffingtonpost.com/entry/thich-nhat-hanh-paris-climate-agreement_us_56a24b7ae4b076aadcc64321, accessed on 25 August 2016.

Costello, A., Mustafa, A., Allen, A., Ball, S. *et al.* (2009) "Managing the health effects of climate change." *Lancet 373*, 1693–1733.

Crowder, N. (2015) "How a small drought town in California's central valley is weathering the state's massive water shortage." *Washington Post*, 15 September 2015. Available at www.washingtonpost.com/news/in-sight/wp/2015/09/15/california-drought-town, accessed on 25 August 2016.

Curfman, G. (ed.) (2009) "Why it's hard to change unhealthy behavior—and why you should keep trying." *Healthbeat: Harvard Health Publications*. Available at www.health.harvard.edu/staying-healthy/why-its-hard-to-change-unhealthy-behavior, accessed on 25 August 2016.

D'Angelo, C. (2016) "Oceans won't have enough oxygen in as little as 15 years." *Grist*, 29 April 2016. Available at http://grist.org/climate-energy/oceans-wont-have-enough-oxygen-in-as-little-as-15-years/?utm_content=bufferff91c&utm_medium=social&utm_source=facebook.com&utm_campaign=buffer, accessed on 25 August 2016.

Danieli, Y. (1984) "Psychotherapists' participation in the conspiracy of silence about the holocaust." *Psychoanalytic Psychology 1*, 23–42.

Darabi, G. (2015) "In your backyard." *Al Jazeera*, 16 December 2015. Available at www.aljazeera.com/programmes/earthrise/2015/12/backyard-151216101228687.html, accessed on 25 August 2016.

Davenport, C. and Robertson, C. (2016) "Resettling the first American 'climate refugees.'" *The New York Times*. Available at www.nytimes.com/2016/05/03/us/resettling-the-first-american-climate-refugees.html?_r=0, accessed on 25 August 2016.

Davenport, L. (2009) *Healing and Transformation Through Self Guided Imagery.* Berkeley, CA: Celestial Arts.

Davenport, L. (ed.) (2016) *Transformative Imagery: Cultivating the Imagination for Healing, Change, and Growth.* London: Jessica Kingsley Publishers.

DeAngelis, T. (2008) "The two faces of oxytocin." *American Psychological Association, Science Watch 39*, 2, 30.

Doherty, T. and Clayton, S. (2011) "The psychological impacts of global climate change." *American Psychologist, 66*, May–June, 265–276.

Doka, K. (ed.) (2002) *Disenfranchised Grief: New Directions, Challenges, and Strategies for Practice.* Champaign, Il: Research Books.

East, S. (2016) "Four years' trash, one jar... zero waste." *CNN*, 6 July 2016. Available at www.cnn.com/2016/07/04/us/lauren-singer-zero-waste-blogger-plastic, accessed on 25 August 2016.

Emmons, R. (2010) "Why gratitude is good." *University of California, Berkeley Greater Good Newsletter*, 16 November 2010. Available at http://greatergood.berkeley.edu/article/item/why_gratitude_is_good, accessed on 25 August 2016.

English, B. (2015) "Proving insights into overcoming disaster." *Boston Globe*, 31 August 2015. Available at www.bostonglobe.com/lifestyle/2015/08/31/resilience/u4TXnte3a9JKNs9D2K7AOO/story.html, accessed on 25 August 2016.

Fan, Y., Duncan, N., de Greck, M., and Northoff, G. (2011) "Is there a core neural network in empathy? An fMRI based quantitative meta-analysis." *Neuroscience and Biobehavioral Review 35*, 903–911.

Federal Emergency Management Agency (1995) "Disaster assistance: A guide to recovery programs." *A Federal Interagency Publication Developed by Signatories to the National Response Plan 229*, 4.

Fehrenbacher, J. (2014) "Iceland's Solheimar ecovillage is still going strong after 84 years." *Inhabitat*. Available at http://inhabitat.com/icelandic-eco-village, accessed on 25 August 2016.

Festinger, L. (1954) "A theory of social comparison processes." *Human Relations 7*, 117–140.

Field, C., Barros, V., Stocker, T., Dahe, Q. *et al.* (eds) (2012) *Managing the Risks of Extreme Events and Disasters to Advance Climate Change Adaptation*. New York, NY: Cambridge University Press. Available at www.ipcc.ch/pdf/special-reports/srex/SREX_Full_Report.pdf, accessed on 25 August 2016.

Finneran, M. (2013) "More extreme weather events forecast." *NASA*, 16 January 2013. Available at www.nasa.gov/centers/langley/science/climate_assessment_2012.html, accessed on 25 August 2016.

Fisher, C. and Garnett, T. (2016) *Plate, Pyramids and Planets: Developments in National Healthy and Sustainable Dietary Guidelines: A State of Play Assessment*. Rome: Food and Agriculture Organization of the United Nations. Available at www.fao.org/3/a-i5640e.pdf, accessed on 25 August 2016.

Fort Worth Water Department (2016) "After more than 24 hours, Fort Worth rescinds boil order notice." *CBS DFW News*, 5 February 2016. Available at http://dfw.cbslocal.com/2016/02/05/no-drinking-from-the-tap-as-the-fort-worth-boil-order-continues, accessed on 25 August 2016.

Friedman, M. (2002) *Capitalism and Freedom: Fortieth Anniversary Edition*. Chicago, IL: The University of Chicago.

Fritz, C. (1996) *Disasters and Mental Health: Therapeutic Principles Drawn from Disaster Studies*. Newark, DE: University of Delaware.

Fyall, J. (2009) "Scientist says warming will 'wipe out billions' if political leaders fail to act." *World News Trust*, 29 November 2009. Available at http://worldnewstrust.com/scientist-says-warming-will-wipe-out-billions-if-political-leaders-fail-to-act-jenny-fyall1876, accessed on 25 August 2016.

Gabel, M. (2015) "Regenerative development: going beyond sustainability." *Kosmos Journal*. Available at www.kosmosjournal.org/article/regenerative-development-going-beyond-sustainability/#comments, accessed on 25 August 2016.

Gardner, A. (2009) "Being near nature improves physical, mental health." *USA Today*, 15 October 2009. Available at http://usatoday30.usatoday.com/news/health/2009-10-15-nature-anxiety-exercise_N.htm, accessed on 25 August 2016.

Garfield, C., Spring, C., and Cahill, S. (1998) *Wisdom Circles: A Guide to Discovery and Community Building in Small Groups*. New York, NY: Hyperion.

Geiling, N. (2015) "California's drought could upend America's entire food system." *Progressive Democrats of America*, 25 May 2015. Available at www.pdamerica.org/issues/stop-global-warming/item/563-california-s-drought-could-upend-america-s-entire-food-system, accessed on 25 August 2016.

Gifford, R., Kormos, C., and McIntyre, A. (2011) "Behavioral dimensions of climate change: drivers, responses, barriers, and interventions." *Wiley Interdisciplinary Reviews: Climate Change 2*, 801–827.

Goetz, J., Keltner, D., and Simon-Thomas, E. (2010) "Compassion: an evolutionary analysis and empirical review." *Psychological Bulletin 136*, 3, 351.

Goodier, R. (2011) "Can open source hardware change how we farm? *Engineering for Change*, 12 May 2011. Available at www.engineeringforchange.org/can-open-source-hardware-change-how-we-farm, accessed on 25 August 2016.

Graham, L. (2013) *Bouncing Back: Rewiring your Brain for Maximum Resilience and Well-Being*. Novato, CA: New World Library.

Graham, R., Finney, M., McHugh, C., Cohen, D. *et al*. (2012) *Fourmile Canyon Fire Findings*. Fort Collins, CO: United States Department of Agriculture/Forest Service Rocky Mountain Research Station.

Gutmann, A. (2007) "The lure and dangers of extremist rhetoric." *The University of Pennsylvania Website*. Available at www.upenn.edu/president/meet-president/extremist-rhetoric, accessed on 25 August 2016.

Hagerman, S., Satterfield, T., and Dowlatabadi, H. (2010) "Climate change impacts, conservation and protected values: understanding promotion, ambivalence and resistance to policy change at the world conservation congress." *Conservation and Society 8*, 4, 298–311.

Hale, C. (2015) "World leaders must listen to Pope Francis on climate change." *Time Magazine*, 2 December 2015. Available at: http://time.com/4132104/paris-climate-conference-pope-francis, accessed on 25 August 2016.

Hall, J. (2016) "Canberra at the centre of a renewable energy superpower." *The Canberra Times*, 23 April 2016. Available at www.canberratimes.com.au/act-news/canberra-at-the-centre-of-a-renewable-energy-superpower-20160422-god1w9.html, accessed on 25 August 2016.

Hamilton, C. (2010) *Requiem for a Species: Why We Resist the Truth About Climate Change*. New York, NY: Taylor and Francis Group.

Hạnh, T. N. (1987) *Interbeing: Fourteen Guidelines for Engaged Buddhism*. Berkeley, CA: Parallax Press.

Hạnh, T. N. and Ellsberg, R. (ed.) (2001) *Thích Nhất Hạnh: Essential Writings*. Maryknoll, NY: Orbis Books.

Happynook, T. (2005) "Securing Nuu Chah Nulth food, health and traditional values through the sustainable use of marine mammals." *Turtle Island Native Network News.* Available at www.turtleisland.org/news/news-Nuuchahnulth.htm, accessed on 25 August 2016.

Harrabin, R. (2015) "Is it ok for scientists to weep over climate change?" *The Guardian,* 9 July 2015. Available at www.theguardian.com/environment/2015/jul/09/is-it-ok-scientists-weep-over-climate-change, accessed on 25 August 2016.

Hawken, P. (2008) *Blessed Unrest: How the Largest Social Movement in History is Restoring Grace, Justice, and Beauty to the World.* New York, NY: Penguin Books.

Heath, C. and Heath, D. (2010) *Switch: How to Change Things When Change is Hard.* New York, NY: Crown Business.

Hernandez-Wolfe, P. (2013) *A Borderlands View on Latinos, Latin Americans, and Decolonization: Rethinking Mental Health.* Lanham, MD: The Rowman and Littlefield Publishing Group.

Hobfoll, S., Watson, P., Bell, C., Bryant, R. *et al.* (2007) "Five essential elements of immediate and mid-term trauma intervention: empirical evidence." *Psychiatry 70,* 4, 283–315.

Hoffman, E. (2013) "When empathy hurts, compassion can heal." *Greater Good in Action.* Berkeley, CA: University of California. Available at http://greatergood. berkeley.edu/article/item/when_empathy_hurts_compassion_can_heal, accessed on 25 August 2016.

Hoggan, J. (2016) *I'm Right and You're an Idiot: The Toxic State of Public Discourse and How to Clean it Up.* Gabriola Island: New Society Publishers.

Holmes, J. (2015) "Climate scientists are dealing with psychological problems." *Science of Us, NYMag,* 9 July 2015. Available at http://nymag.com/science ofus/2015/07/climate-scientists-face-psychological-problems.html, accessed on 25 August 2016.

Howell, E. (2014) "How many galaxies are there?" *Space.com,* 1 April 2014. Available at www.space.com/25303-how-many-galaxies-are-in-the-universe.html, accessed on 25 August 2016.

Husted, K. (2012) "Seattle's first urban food forest will be open to foragers." *National Public Radio,* 1 March 2012. Available at www.npr.org/sections/ thesalt/2012/02/29/147668557/seattles-first-urban-food-forest-will-be-free-to-forage, accessed on 25 August 2016.

Jacobson, M. and Delucchi, M. (2009) "A plan to power 100 percent of the planet with renewables." *Scientific American,* 1 November 2009. Available at www. scientificamerican.com/article.cfm?id=a-path-to-sustainable-energy-by-2030, accessed on 25 August 2016.

Jacobson, M. and Delucchi, M. (2011) "Providing all global energy with wind, water, and solar power, part II: reliability, system and transmission costs, and policies." *Energy Policy 39,* 1170–1190.

Jarero, I., Artigas, L., and Montero, M. (2008) "The EMDR integrative group treatment protocol: application with child victims of mass disaster." *Journal of EMDR Practice and Research 2,* 97–105.

Jedlicka, W. (2010) *Sustainable Graphic Design: Tools, Systems and Strategies for Innovative Print Design.* Hoboken, NJ: John Wiley and Sons.

Johnston, I. (2016) "Rate of species decline 'no longer within safe limit' for humans, experts warn." *Independent,* 14 July 2016 Available at www.independent.co.uk/environment/extinct-species-biodiversity-loss-ecosystems-anthropocene-journal-science-a7137476.html, accessed on 25 August 2016.

Jones, S. (2016) "World heading for catastrophe over natural disasters, risk expert warns." *The Guardian,* 24 April 2016. Available at www.theguardian.com/global-development/2016/apr/24/world-heading-for-catastrophe-over-natural-disasters-risk-expert-warns, accessed on 25 August 2016.

Kabat-Zinn, J., Massion, A., Kristeller, J., and Peterson, L. (1992) "Effectiveness of a meditation-based stress reduction program in the treatment of anxiety disorders." *American Journal of Psychiatry 149,* 936–943.

Kahan, D., Peters, E., Wittlin, M., Slovic, P. *et al.* (2012) "The polarizing impact of science literacy and numeracy on perceived climate change risks." *Nature Climate Change Letters 1547.* Available at www.climateaccess.org/sites/default/files/Kahan_Polarizing%20Impact%20of%20Science%20Literacy.pdf, accessed on 25 August 2016.

Kahn, B. (2016) "Antarctic CO2 hits 400 ppm for first time in 4 million years." *Climate Central,* 15 June 2016. Available at www.climatecentral.org/news/antarctica-co2-400-ppm-million-years-20451, accessed on 25 August 2016.

Karl, T., Melillo, J., and Peterson, T. (eds) (2009) *Global Climate Change Impacts in the United States.* New York, NY: Cambridge University Press.

Kassinove, H. and Tafrate, R. (2002) *Anger Management: The Complete Treatment Guidebook for Practitioners.* Atascadero, CA: Impact Publishers.

Keefe, S. (2014) "This Canadian artist halted pipeline development by copyrighting his land as a work of art." *Vice,* 6 November 2014. Available at www.vice.com/read/this-canadian-artist-halted-pipeline-development-by-copyrighting-his-land-as-a-work-of-art-983, accessed on 25 August 2016.

Keefer, M, (2013) "Noam Chomsky: indigenous people are in the lead." *Popular Resistance,* 9 November 2013. Available at www.popularresistance.org/noam-chomsky-indigenous-people-are-in-the-lead, accessed on 25 August 2016.

Keller, H. (1933) "The simplest way to be happy." *Home Magazine 7,* 2, 6.

Keltner, D., Marsh, J., and Smith, J. (eds) (2010) *The Compassionate Instinct: The Science of Human Goodness.* New York, NY: WW Norton and Company.

Key, R. (2016) "Boil water advisory affecting most of Augusta Georgia will last into Thursday." *WJBF 6 News,* 9 February 2016. Available at http://wjbf.com/2016/02/09/thousands-affected-by-augusta-boil-water-advisory, accessed on 25 August 2016.

Kini, P., Wong, J., McInnis, S., Gabana, N. *et al.* (2016) "The effects of gratitude expression on neural activity." *Neuroimage 128,* 1–10.

Klausner, S. and Kincaid, H. (1956) *Social Problems of Sheltering Flood Victims.* New York, NY: Bureau of Applied Social Research, Columbia University.

Klein, H. (ed.) (1968) *Massive Psychic Trauma*. New York, NY: International Universities Press.

Klein, N. (2007) *The Shock Doctrine: The Rise of Disaster Capitalism*. New York, NY: Henry Holt and Company.

Klein, N. (2014) "If black lives mattered…" *The Nation*, 16 December 2014. Available at www.thenation.com/article/if-black-lives-mattered, accessed on 25 August 2016.

Klimecki, O., Leiberg, S., Lamm, C., and Singer, T. (2013) "Functional neural plasticity and associated changes in positive affect after compassion training." *Cerebral Cortex 23*, 7, 1552–1561.

Knieling, J. and Filho, W. (2012) *Climate Change Governance*. New York, NY: Springer.

Kolb, D. (2014) *Experiential Learning: Experience as the Source of Learning and Development*. 2nd edition. Upper Saddle River, NJ: Pearson Education.

Kolbert, E. (2014) *The Sixth Extinction: An Unnatural History*. New York, NY: Henry Holt and Company.

Kolbert, E. (2015) "The weight of the world: can Christiana Figueres persuade humanity to save itself?" *The New Yorker*, 24 August 2015. Available at www.newyorker.com/magazine/2015/08/24/the-weight-of-the-world, accessed on 25 August 2016.

Kouzes, J. and Posner, B. (1999) *Encouraging the Heart: A Leader's Guide to Rewarding and Recognizing Others*. San Francisco, CA: Jossey-Bass Publishers.

Kroh, K. (2013) "After the flood: how climate change changed one Colorado community forever." *ThinkProgress*, 10 October 2013. Available at http://thinkprogress.org/climate/2013/10/10/2741901/colorado-flood-fire, accessed on 25 August 2016.

Krystal, B. (2015) "How to find shrimp that's not produced by slave labor in Thailand." *The Washington Post*, 16 December 2015. Available at www.washingtonpost.com/news/food/wp/2015/12/16/how-to-find-shrimp-thats-not-produced-by-slave-labor-in-thailand, accessed on 25 August 2016.

Landau, J. (2007) "Enhancing resilience: families and communities as agents for change." *Family Process 46*, 3, 351–365.

Leaning, J. and Guha-Sapir, D. (2013) "Natural disasters, armed conflict, and public health." *New England Journal of Medicine 369*, 1836–1842.

Leiserowitz, A., Maibach, E., Roser-Renouf, C., Feinberg, G., and Rosenthal, S. (2015) *Climate Change in the American Mind*. New Haven, CT: Yale Project on Climate Change Communication and George Mason University Center for Climate Change Communication. Available at http://environment.yale.edu/climate-communication/files/Global-Warming-CCAM-March-2015.pdf, accessed on 25 August 2016.

LeMay, K. (2016) "Social change and unfelt heartbreak." *Linkedin Pulse*, 15 January 2016. Available at www.linkedin.com/pulse/social-change-unfelt-heartbreak-kathy-lemay, accessed on 25 August 2016.

Lertzman, R. (2015) "In climate change, psychology often gets lost in translation." *Pacific Standard*, 24 November 2015. Available at www.psmag.com/nature-and-technology/in-climate-change-psychology-often-gets-lost-in-translation, accessed on 25 August 2016.

Levine, P. (1997) *Waking the Tiger: Healing Trauma*. Berkeley, CA: North Atlantic Books.

Lynn, K., MacKendrick, K., and Donoghue, E. (2011) *Social Vulnerability and Climate Change: A Synthesis of Literature*. Portland, OR: U.S. Department of Agriculture.

Macy, J. and Brown, M. (2014) *Coming Back to Life: The Guide to the Work that Reconnects*. Gabriola Island: New Society Publishers.

Macy, J. and Johnstone, C. (2012) *Active Hope: How to Face the Mess We're in without Going Crazy*. Novato, CA: New World Library.

Maguen, S. and Litz, B. (2015) "Moral injury in the context of war." *U.S. Department of Veterans Affairs*. Available at www.ptsd.va.gov/professional/co-occurring/moral_injury_at_war.asp, accessed on 25 August 2016.

Mallapur, C. (2015) "61% rise in heat-stroke deaths over decade." *IndiaSpend*, 27 May 2015. Available at www.indiaspend.com/cover-story/61-rise-in-heat-stroke-deaths-over-decade-60404, accessed on 25 August 2016.

Maller, C., Townsend, M., Pryor, A., Brown, P., and St. Leger, L. (2005) "Healthy nature healthy people: 'contact with nature' as an upstream health promotion intervention for populations." *Oxford Journals 21*, 1, 45–54.

Mandel, C. (2015) "Bill McKibben: 'Canada is an obstructive and dangerous force upon the planet.'" *National Observer*, 2 July 2015 Available at www.nationalobserver.com/2015/07/02/news/bill-mckibben-canada-obstructive-and-dangerous-force-upon-planet, accessed on 25 August 2016.

Marshall, C., Bush, D., Smalls, M., Stafford, E. *et al.* (2012) Climate Change, Environmental Challenges and Vulnerable Communities: Assessing Legacies of the Past, Building Opportunities for the Future. Washington, DC: Joint Center for Political and Economic Studies. Available at http://jointcenter.org/sites/default/files/Joint%20Center%20Climate%20Change%2C%20Environmental%20Challenges%20and%20Vulnerable%20Communities%20Report.pdf, accessed on 25 August 2016.

Massachusetts Department of Environmental Protection (2016) "MassDEP drinking water program: public health orders." *Massachusetts Department of Environmental Protection*. Available at http://public.dep.state.ma.us/boil_order, accessed on 25 August 2016.

McDonough, P. (2009) "TV viewing among kids at an eight-year high." *The Nielsen Company*. Available at www.nielsen.com/us/en/insights/news/2009/tv-viewing-among-kids-at-an-eight-year-high.html, accessed on 19 September 2016.

McKibben, B. (2013) *Oil and Honey: The Education of an Unlikely Activist*. New York, NY: Times Books.

McLeod, H. (2015) "South Carolina hit by torrential rainfall, eight dead." *Reuters*, 5 October 2015. Available at www.reuters.com/article/us-usa-weather-floods-idUSKCN0RY0RJ20151005, accessed on 25 August 2016.

Mena-Werth, R. (2016) "Scientists suggest appealing to human psychology to create solutions to climate change." *Stanford News*, 13 April 2016. Available at http://news.stanford.edu/2016/04/13/scientists-suggest-appealing-human-psychology-create-solutions-climate-change, accessed on 25 August 2016.

Mercer, G. (2016) "The link between zika and climate change." *The Atlantic*, 24 February 2016. Available at www.theatlantic.com/health/archive/2016/02/zika-and-climate-change/470643, accessed on 25 August 2016.

Mitchell, D. (2015) "How toxic algae is ruining the crab season." *Fortune*, 18 December 2015. Available at http://fortune.com/2015/12/18/toxic-algae-crab-sea-lion, accessed on 25 August 2016.

Mitchell, J. (1983) "When disaster strikes...the critical incident stress debriefing process." *Journal of Emergency Medical Services 13*, 11, 49–52.

Mittal, A. (2005) "Lake Pontchartrain and vicinity hurricane protection project." *Army Corp of Engineers*. Washington DC: GAO.

Mobbs, D., Hagan, C., Dalgleish, T., Silton, B., and Prevost, C. (2015) "The ecology of human fear: survival optimization and the nervous system." *Frontiers in Neuroscience 9*, 55.

Mullen, J. (2015) "Downpour floods parts of the French Riviera: at least 20 dead." *CNN*, 5 October 2015. Available at www.cnn.com/2015/10/04/europe/france-french-riviera-flooding, accessed on 25 August 2016.

Mulvihill, J. (2010) "Katrina five years after: hurricane left a legacy of health concerns." *Fox News*, 27 August 2010. Available at www.foxnews.com/story/2010/08/27/katrina-five-years-after-hurricane-left-legacy-health-concerns.html, accessed on 25 August 2016.

National Wildlife Federation (2008) Increased Risk of Catastrophic Wild Fires: Global Warming's Wake Up Call for the Western United States. Merrifield, VA: National Wildlife Federation. Available at www.nwf.org/~/media/PDFs/Global-Warming/NWF_WildFiresFinal.ashx, accessed on 25 August 2016.

New Hampshire Department of Environmental Services (2016) "Drinking water advisories." *Drinking Water and Underground Bureau*. Available at www2.des.state.nh.us/Advisories/Drinking_Water, accessed on 25 August 2016.

Nin, A. (1972) *Seduction of the Minotaur*. Chicago, IL: The Swallow Press.

NOAA (2013) "Visualizing the September 2013 Colorado flood." *National Centers for Environmental Information*. Available at www.ncdc.noaa.gov/news/visualizing-september-2013-colorado-flood, accessed on 25 August 2016.

Norris, F. H., Friedman, M. J., Watson, P. J., Byrne, C .M., Diaz, E., and Kaniasty, K. (2002) "60,000 disaster victims speak: Part I. An empirical review of the empirical literature, 1981–2001." *Psychiatry 65*, 207–239.

Nutt, D. (2004) "Anxiety and depression: individual entities or two sides of the same coin?" *International Journal of Psychiatry in Clinical Practice 8*, 1, 19–24.

Ohio Environmental Protection Agency (2016) "Current drinking water advisories for Ohio public water systems." *Ohio EPA*. Available at wwwapp.epa.ohio.gov/ddagw/Advisories/advisories.html, accessed on 25 August 2016.

Ohlson, K. (2014) *The Soil Will Save Us: How Scientists, Farmers and Foodies Are Healing the Soil to Save the Planet.* Emmaus, PA: Rodale Books.

Oliver, M. (1992) *New and Selected Poems.* Boston, MA: Beacon Press.

Pachamama Alliance (2016) *Game Changer Intensive: Training Program, Course Handout.* San Francisco, CA: Pachamama Alliance.

Payne, P., Levine, P., and Crane-Godreau, M. (2015) "Somatic experiencing: using interoception and proprioception as core elements of trauma therapy." *Frontiers of Psychology 6,* 1–18.

Pearlman, L. and Saakvitne, K. (1995) *Trauma and the Therapist: Countertransference and Vicarious Traumatization in Psychotherapy with Incest Survivors.* New York, NY: WW Norton and Company.

Pennebaker, J. and Harber, L. (1993) "A social stage model of collective coping: the Loma Prieta earthquake and the Persian Gulf war." *Journal of Social Issues 49,* 125–142.

Penner, D. (2013) "'This town was almost blown off the map—now it's back, and super green." *Grist,* 2 April 2013. Available at http://grist.org/cities/this-town-was-almost-blown-off-the-map-now-its-back-and-super-green, accessed on 25 August 2016.

Petras, K. and Petras R. (2009) *Don't Forget to Sing in the Lifeboats.* New York, NY: Workman Publishing Company.

Phillips, A. (2015) "Denmark sets world record for wind power production." *ThinkProgress,* 7 January 2015. Available at http://thinkprogress.org/climate/2015/01/07/3608898/denmark-sets-world-record-for-wind-power, accessed on 25 August 2016.

Plait, P. (2016) "No human alive has seen 7 months this hot before." *Grist,* 17 May 2016. Available at http://grist.org/climate-energy/no-human-alive-has-seen-7-months-this-hot-before, accessed on 25 August 2016.

Platt, B., Ciplet, D., Bailey, K., and Lombardi, E. (2008) *Stop Trashing the Climate.* Washington DC: Institute for Local Self Reliance.

Pohl, C. (2012) *Living into Community: Cultivating Practices that Sustain Us.* Grand Rapids, MI: Wm. B. Eerdmans Publishing Company.

Pope Francis (2015) "On care for our common home." *Encyclical.* Available at http://w2.vatican.va/content/francesco/en/encyclicals/documents/papa-francesco_20150524_enciclica-laudato-si.html, accessed on 25 August 2016.

Popova, M. (2015) "Some thoughts on hope, cynicism, and the stories we tell ourselves." *Brain Pickings.* Available at www.brainpickings.org/2015/02/09/hope-cynicism, accessed on 25 August 2016.

Popovitch, T. (2014) "10 American cities lead the way with urban agriculture ordinances." *Seedstock,* 27 May 2014. Available at http://seedstock.com/2014/05/27/10-american-cities-lead-the-way-with-urban-agriculture-ordinances, accessed on 25 August 2016.

Post, R., Weiss S., Smith, M., Li, H., and McCann, U. (1997) "Kindling versus quenching: implications for the evolution and treatment of posttraumatic stress disorder." *Annals of the New York Academy of Sciences 821,* 285–295.

Powell, P. and Smith, M. (2011) *"Domestic Violence: An Overview, Fact Sheet-11-76.* Reno, NV: University of Nevada Cooperative Extension. Available at www.unce. unr.edu/publications/files/cy/2011/fs1176.pdf, accessed on 25 August 2016.

Rappaport, L. (2014) *Mindfulness and the Art Therapies: Theory and Practice.* London: Jessica Kingsley Publishers.

Richardson, J. (2015) "When the end of human civilization is your day job." *Esquire,* 7 July 2015. Available at www.esquire.com/news-politics/a36228/ballad-of-the-sad-climatologists-0815, accessed on 25 August 2016.

Riffkin, R. (2014) "Climate change not a top worry in U.S." *Gallup,* 12 March 2014. Available at www.gallup.com/poll/167843/climate-change-not-top-worry.aspx, accessed on 25 August 2016.

Ripley, A. (2009) *The Unthinkable: Who Survives when Disaster Strikes—and Why.* New York, NY: Three Rivers Press.

Robine, J., Cheung, S., Le Roy, S., Van Oyen, H. *et al.* (2008) "Death toll exceeded 70,000 in Europe during the summer of 2003." *Comptes Rendus Biologies 331,* 2, 171–178.

Roewe, B. (2015) "Psychological barriers complicate overcoming climate change denial." *The National Catholic Reporter,* 1 June 2015. Available at http://ncronline. org/blogs/eco-catholic/psychological-barriers-complicate-overcoming-climate-change-denial, accessed on 25 August 2016.

Rothschild, B. (2006) *Help for the Helper: The Psychophysiology of Compassion Fatigue and Vicarious Trauma.* New York, NY: WW Norton and Company.

Running, S. (2007) "Five stages of climate grief." *Numerical Terradynamic Simulation Group, University of Montana,* 26 November 2007. Available at www.ntsg.umt. edu/files/5StagesClimateGrief.htm, accessed on 25 August 2016.

Saad, L. and Jones, J. (2016) "U.S. concern about global warming at eight-year high." *Gallup Poll,* 22 March 2016. Available at http://ecoaffect.org/2016/03/22/new-record-65-of-americans-believe-climate-change-is-caused-by-human-activity, accessed on 25 August 2016.

Sabatini, J. (2016) "SF to require rooftop solar instillations on new buildings." *San Francisco Examiner,* 25 August 2016. Available at www.sfexaminer.com/san-francisco-require-rooftop-solar-installations-new-buildings, accessed on 25 August 2016.

Safransky, S. (1990) *Sunbeams: A Book of Quotations.* Berkeley, CA: North Atlantic Books.

Samenow, J. (2015) "Freak storm in North Atlantic to lash UK, may push temperatures over 50 degrees above normal at North Pole." *The Washington Post,* 28 December 2015. Available at www.washingtonpost.com/news/capital-weather-gang/wp/2015/12/28/freak-storm-in-north-atlantic-may-push-temperatures-70-degrees-above-normal-at-north-pole/?sdfsfdsdfdsf, accessed on 25 August 2016.

Sandler, K. and David, L. (2011) *The Benefits and Challenges of Green Roofs on Public and Commercial Buildings.* Washington, DC: The U.S. General Services Administration. Available at www.gsa.gov/portal/mediaId/158783/fileName/The_Benefits_and_Challenges_of_Green_Roofs_on_Public_and_Commercial_Buildings.action, accessed on 25 August 2016.

Scheer, R. and Moss, D. (2011) "External medicine: discarded drugs may contaminate 40 million Americans' drinking water." *Scientific American*. Available at www. scientificamerican.com/article/pharmaceuticals-in-the-water, accessed on 25 August 2016.

Schroeder, H. (1991) "Preference and meaning of arboretum landscapes: Combining quantitative and qualitative data." *Journal of Environmental Psychology 11*, 231–248.

Schultz, S., Doust, M., Marinello, M., Russell, B., Vines, K., and Zekri, A. (2014) *City of Cleveland*. London: Carbon Disclosure Project.

Scott, B. (2012) "The story of the two wolves: managing your thoughts, feelings and actions." *Psychology Matters—Asia*, 21 February 2012. Available at www. psychologymatters.asia/article/65/the-story-of-the-two-wolves-managing-your-thoughts-feelings-and-actions.html, accessed on 25 August 2016.

Seaward, L. (2011) *Managing Stress: A Creative Journal*. Sudbury, MA: Jones and Bartlett Learning.

Seide, J. (2016) Personal communication and website. Available at www. centerforcouncil.org, accessed on 25 August 2016.

Shapiro, D. (1982) "Overview: clinical and physiological comparison of meditation with other self-control strategies." *American Journal of Psychiatry 139*, 267–274.

Sher, A. (2014) "The gift economy: The model for a collaborative community." *Tikkun*. Available at www.tikkun.org/nextgen/the-gift-economy-a-model-for-collaborative-community, accessed on 25 August 2016.

Siegel, D. (2012) *The Developing Mind: How Relationships and the Brain Interact to Shape Who We Are*. New York, NY: Guilford Press.

Skelton, R. and Miller, V. (2016) "The environmental justice movement." *Natural Resources Defense Council*, 17 March 2016. Available at www.nrdc.org/ej/history/hej.asp, accessed on 25 August 2016.

Smith, H. (2015a) "People are still living in FEMA's toxic trailers—and they likely have no idea." *Grist*, 27 August 2015. Available at http://grist.org/politics/people-are-still-living-in-femas-toxic-katrina-trailers-and-they-likely-have-no-idea, accessed on 25 August 2016.

Smith, T. (2015b) "5 countries leading the way toward 100% renewable energy." *EcoWatch*, 9 January 2015. Available at http://ecowatch.com/2015/01/09/countries-leading-way-renewable-energy, accessed on 25 August 2016.

Smith, R. (2015c) "How reducing food waste could ease climate change." *National Geographic*, 22 January 2015. Available at http://news.nationalgeographic.com/news/2015/01/150122-food-waste-climate-change-hunger, accessed on 25 August 2016.

Snodgrass, W. (2002) *To Sound Like Yourself: Essays on Poetry*. Rochester, NY: BOA Editions, Ltd.

Solnit, R. (2009) *A Paradise Built in Hell: The Extraordinary Communities that Arise in Disaster*. New York, NY: Viking Penguin.

Sonnentag, S. and Zijlstra, F. (2006) "Job characteristics and off-job activities as predictors of need for recovery, well-being, and fatigue." *Journal of Applied Psychology 91*, 2, 330–350.

Sprenkle, D. and Piercy, F. (eds) (2005) *Research Methods in Family Therapy.* New York, NY: Guilford Press.

Stamm, B. (1997) "Work-related secondary traumatic stress." *PTSD Research Quarterly 8*, 25–34.

Stoknes, P. E. (2014) "Rethinking climate communications and the psychological climate paradox." *Energy Research and Social Science 1*, 161–170.

Sutter, J. (2015) "Why beef is the new SUV." *CNN News*, 25 November 2015. Available at www.cnn.com/2015/09/29/opinions/sutter-beef-suv-cliamte-two-degrees, accessed on 25 August 2016.

Suzuki, S. (2006) *Zen Mind, Beginner's Mind.* Boston, MA: Shambhala Publications.

Swimme, B. (2007) "Swimme 10: being responsible." *YouTube.* Available at www.youtube.com/watch?v=I8ZcSw1KOSM, accessed on 25 August 2016.

Tannen, D. (1999) *The Argument Culture: Stopping America's War of Words.* New York, NY: Ballantine Books.

Tapsell, S. and Tunstall, S. M. (2008) "I wish I'd never heard of Banbury: the relationship between 'place' and the health impacts of flooding." *Health & Place 14*, 2, 133–154.

Tatham, H. and Gaffney, A. (2016) "Food street: feeding off the kerbside and creating close communities." *ABS News*, 22 April 2016. Available at www.abc.net.au/news/2016-04-22/food-street-feeding-off-the-kerbside-creates-close-community/7343456, accessed on 25 August 2016.

Taylor, S. and Brown, J. (1988) "Illusion and well-being: A psychosocial perspective on mental health." *American Psychological Association Bulletin 103*, 2, 193–210.

Taylor, S., Klein, L., Lewis, B., Gruenewald, T., Gurung, R., and Updegraff, J. (2000) "Biobehavioral responses to stress in females: Tend-and-befriend, not fight-or-flight." *Psychological Review 107*, 3, 411–429.

The Economist (2007) "The slow recovery: two years after Katrina, New Orleans is still a shadow of its past self. *The Economist*, 23 August 2007. Available at www.economist.com/node/9687404, accessed on 25 August 2016.

Thiele, L. (2013) *Indra's Net and the Midas Touch.* Cambridge. MA: The MIT Press.

Thomas, M. (2014) "Climate depression is for real: just ask a scientist." *Grist*, 28 October 2014. Available at http://grist.org/climate-energy/climate-depression-is-for-real-just-ask-a-scientist, accessed on 25 August 2016.

Thomas, M. (2016) "We're inching closer to making solar power as cheap as regular electricity." *Pacific Standard*. Available at https://psmag.com/were-inching-closer-to-making-solar-power-as-cheap-as-regular-electricity-d1fe298d189f#.br4efo6ql, accessed on 25 August 2016.

Thomas, H. and Thomas M. (2013) *Economics for People and Earth: The Auroville Case 1968–2008.* Tamil Nadu: Social Research Center.

Town of Jamestown (2013) "Jamestown 2013 flood facts." *Jamestownco.org.* Available at www.jamestownco.org/jamestown-2013-flood-facts, accessed on 25 August 2016.

Ulrich, R., Simons, R., Losito, B., Fiorito, E., Miles, M., and Zelson, M. (1991) "Stress recovery during exposure to natural and urban environments." *Journal of Environmental Psychology 113*, 3, 201–230.

United Way (2014) "New flood mental health voucher fact sheet." *Foothills United Way.* Available at http://bocofloodrecovery.org/wp-content/uploads/2014/01/voucherFACTsheet.pdf, accessed on 25 August 2016.

Van Susteren, L. (2011) "Our moral obligation." *Huffington Post*, 25 May 2011. Available at www.huffingtonpost.com/lise-van-susteren/our-moral-obligation_b_187751.html, accessed on 25 August 2016.

Van Zomeren, M., Spears, R., and Leach, C. (2010) "Experimental evidence for a dual pathway model analysis of coping with the climate crisis." *Journal of Environmental Psychology 30*, 4, 339–346.

Vidal, J. (2013) "UK vineyards enjoy bumper crop in 'perfect year.'" *The Guardian*, 2 August 2013. Available at www.theguardian.com/lifeandstyle/2013/aug/02/vineyards-bumper-crop-perfect-year, accessed on 25 August 2016.

Vujanovic, A., Youngwirth, N., Johnson, K., and Zvolensky, M. (2009) "Mindfulness-based acceptance and posttraumatic stress symptoms among trauma-exposed adults without axis I psychopathology." *Journal of Anxiety Disorders 23*, 297–303.

Walsh, F. (2007) "Traumatic loss and major disasters: strengthening family and community resilience." *Family Process 46*, 2, 207–227.

Washington State Department of Health (2016) "Recent drinking water alerts." *Community and Environment Recent Alerts.* Available at www.doh.wa.gov/CommunityandEnvironment/DrinkingWater/Alerts/RecentAlerts, accessed on 25 August 2016.

Weissbecker, I. (ed.) (2011) *Climate Change and Human Well-Being: Global Challenges and Opportunities.* New York, NY: Springer.

Werber, C. (2016) "Al Gore is hugely optimistic when it comes to one thing about climate change." *Quartz*, 15 April 2016. Available at http://qz.com/662233/al-gore-is-hugely-optimistic-when-it-comes-to-one-thing-about-climate-change, accessed on 25 August 2016.

West Virginia American Water (2016) "Boil water orders." *The Register Herald*, 14 May 2016. Available at www.register-herald.com/news/boil-water-orders/article_21d03de3-5527-590f-98db-092fe2c34694.html, accessed on 25 August 2016.

Whyte, D. (2015) *Consolations: The Solace, Nourishment and Underlying Meaning of Everyday Words.* Langley, WA: Many Rivers Press.

Winn, P. (2015) "The slave labor behind your favorite clothing brands: Gap, H&M and more exposed." *Salon*, 22 March 2015. Available at www.salon.com/2015/03/22/the_slave_labor_behind_your_favorite_clothing_brands_gap_hm_and_more_exposed_partner, accessed on 25 August 2016.

World Health Organization (2016) *WHO Global Urban Ambient Air Pollution Database*. Geneva: World Health Organization. Available at www.who.int/phe/ health_topics/outdoorair/databases/cities/en, accessed on 25 August 2016.

Yes! Magazine (2016) "No fossil fuel? No problem—7 ways we're already living more locally." *Yes! Magazine*, 11 April 2016. Available at www.yesmagazine.org/issues/ life-after-oil/no-fossil-fuel-no-problem-7-ways-were-already-living-more-locally-20160411, accessed on 25 August 2016.

Young, B., Ford, J., Ruzek, J., Friedman, M., and Gusman, F. (1998) *Disaster Mental Health Services: A Guidebook for Clinicians and Administrators*. White River Junction, VT: The National Center for Post-Traumatic Stress Disorder Education and Clinical Laboratory, Executive Divisions VA Palo Alto Health Care System, VA Medical & Regional Office Center White River Junction.

Zeller, T. (2010) "Failed efforts in protecting biodiversity." *The New York Times*, 31 January 2010. Available at www.nytimes.com/2010/02/01/business/ global/01green.html?pagewanted=all&_r=1, accessed on 25 August 2016.

Zia, A. and Waddick. C. (2015) "Climate policy needs a new vision." *Sci Dev Net*, 14 October 2015. Available at www.scidev.net/global/opinion/climate-change-policy-vision-unfccc.html#sthash.A9NUKMuh.dpu, accessed on 25 August 2016.

Zimmerman, J. and Coyle, V. (2009) *The Way of Council*. Viroqua, WI: Bramble Books.

NOTES

Part I

CHAPTER 1

1. www.pachamama.org/engage/awakening-the-dreamer
2. Excerpted and modified from the motivational interviewing mode: Sobell, L. C. and Sobell, M. B. (2008) Motivational Interviewing Strategies and Techniques: Rationales and Examples. Available at www.nova.edu/gsc/forms/mi_rationale_ techniques.pdf, accessed on 25 August 2016.

CHAPTER 2

1. The field of psychology sees a difference between emotions and feelings. An emotion is physically based, a hardwired psychological reaction, and it precedes feelings. Feelings are the conscious awareness of the emotion, and they become tied to beliefs. It is possible to change feelings as our life experience grows. While this distinction is important, in this book the terms are used more fluidly.
2. While this story is generally attributed to Cherokee legend, the origins are undocumented and have been disputed.
3. A free downloadable mp3 recording of this practice can be found at lesliedavenport.com

CHAPTER 3

1. The details of Amy's story, including her name, have been altered and composites employed to protect client confidentiality.

2. A new website, Climate Signals, is taking a scientific look at linking extreme weather events with climate change. It can be accessed at www.climatesignals.org

3. A free downloadable mp3 recording of this practice can be found at www.lesliedavenport.com

CHAPTER 4

1. The original protocol for the Butterfly Hug method is available at http://emdrresearchfoundation.org/toolkit/butterfly-hug.pdf

CHAPTER 5

1. A free, downloadable mp3 of Peaceful Place and Forgiveness Meditation is available at www.lesliedavenport.com

2. A free, downloadable mp3 of Peaceful Place and Forgiveness Meditation is available at www.lesliedavenport.com

CHAPTER 6

1. A free downloadable mp3 recording of this practice can be found at www.lesliedavenport.com

Part II

1. See: www.youtube.com/watch?v=3l5trL3MLIc
2. See: www.youtube.com/watch?v=kHnRIAVXTMQ
3. See: www.youtube.com/watch?v=uoYsQnENTUM

APPENDIX

1. A free, downloadable mp3 recording of this practice can be found at www.lesliedavenport.com

Subject Index

Author Index